Foot and Ankle Osteotomies

Editor

CHRISTOPHER F. HYER

CLINICS IN PODIATRIC MEDICINE AND SURGERY

www.podiatric.theclinics.com

Consulting Editor
THOMAS ZGONIS

July 2015 • Volume 32 • Number 3

ELSEVIER

1600 John F. Kennedy Boulevard • Suite 1800 • Philadelphia, Pennsylvania, 19103-2899

http://www.theclinics.com

CLINICS IN PODIATRIC MEDICINE AND SURGERY Volume 32, Number 3
July 2015 ISSN 0891-8422, ISBN-13: 978-0-323-39115-3

Editor: Jennifer Flynn-Briggs
Developmental Editor: Casey Jackson

Clinics in Podiatric Medicine and Surgery (ISSN 0891-8422) is published quarterly by Elsevier Inc., 360 Park Avenue South, New York, NY 10010-1710. Months of issue are January, April, July, and October. Business and Editorial Offices: 1600 John F. Kennedy Blvd., Ste. 1800, Philadelphia, PA 19103-2899. Customer Service Office: 3251 Riverport Lane, Maryland Heights, MO 63043. Periodicals postage paid at New York, NY and additional mailing offices. Subscription prices are $305.00 per year for US individuals, $450.00 per year for US institutions, $155.00 per year for US students and residents, $370.00 per year for Canadian individuals, $544.00 for Canadian institutions, $435.00 for international individuals, $544.00 per year for international institutions and $220.00 per year for Canadian and foreign students/residents. To receive student/resident rate, orders must be accompanied by name of affiliated institution, date of term, and the *signature* of program/residency coordinator on institution letterhead. Orders will be billed at individual rate until proof of status is received. Foreign air speed delivery is included in all *Clinics* subscription prices. All prices are subject to change without notice. POSTMASTER: Send address changes to *Clinics in Podiatric Medicine and Surgery*, Elsevier Health Sciences Division, Subscription Customer Service, 3251 Riverport Lane, Maryland Heights, MO 63043. **Customer Service: 1-800-654-2452 (US). From outside of the US, call 314-447-8871. Fax: 314-447-8029. E-mail: JournalsCustomerService-usa@elsevier.com (for print support); JournalsOnlineSupport-usa@elsevier.com (for online support).**

Reprints. For copies of 100 or more of articles in this publication, please contact the Commercial Reprints Department, Elsevier Inc., 360 Park Avenue South, New York, NY 10010-1710. Tel.: 212-633-3874; Fax: 212-633-3820; E-mail: reprints@elsevier.com.

Clinics in Podiatric Medicine and Surgery is covered in *MEDLINE/PubMed (Index Medicus)* and *EMBASE/Excerpta Medica*.

CLINICS IN PODIATRIC MEDICINE AND SURGERY

CONSULTING EDITOR
THOMAS ZGONIS, DPM, FACFAS

Contributors

CONSULTING EDITOR

THOMAS ZGONIS, DPM, FACFAS
Professor and Director, Externship and Reconstructive Foot and Ankle Fellowship
Programs, Division of Podiatric Medicine and Surgery, Department of Orthopedics,
University of Texas Health Science Center San Antonio, San Antonio, Texas

EDITOR

CHRISTOPHER F. HYER, DPM, MS, FACFAS
Co-Director, Foot and Ankle Surgery Fellowship, Orthopedic Foot and Ankle Center;
Residency Director, Podiatric Medicine and Surgery Residency, Grant Medical Center,
Columbus, Ohio

AUTHORS

THOMAS C. BEIDEMAN, DPM
PGY-3, Mercy Suburban Hospital, Norristown, Pennsylvania

STEPHEN A. BRIGIDO, DPM, FACFAS
Foot and Ankle Department, Coordinated Health, Bethlehem, Pennsylvania

DEVON CONSUL, BSN, RN
D.P.M. Candidate, Dr. William M. Scholl College of Podiatric Medicine, North Chicago,
Illinois

JAMES M. COTTOM, DPM, FACFAS
Fellowship Director, Attending Physician, Coastal Orthopedics and Sports Medicine,
Bradenton, Florida

WILLIAM T. DECARBO, DPM, FACFAS
The Orthopedic Group, Pittsburgh, Pennsylvania

PREMJIT PETE S. DEOL, DO
Orthopaedics Department, Panorama Orthopedics and Spine Center, Golden, Colorado

J. GEORGE DEVRIES, DPM, FACFAS
Foot and Ankle Surgeon, Orthopedics and Sports Medicine, BayCare Clinic, Manitowoc;
Green Bay, Wisconsin

LINDA FERRAZ, MD
Nimes, France

MELISSA M. GALLI, DPM, MHA, AACFAS
Attending Physician, Department of Orthopedics, The CORE Institute, Phoenix,
Arizona

BRIAN GRADISEK, DPM, AACFAS
Fellow, Weil Foot and Ankle Institute, Chicago, Illinois

CHRISTOPHER F. HYER, DPM, MS, FACFAS
Co-Director, Foot and Ankle Surgery Fellowship, Orthopedic Foot and Ankle Center;
Residency Director, Podiatric Medicine and Surgery Residency, Grant Medical Center,
Columbus, Ohio

JULIEN LABORDE, MD
Clinique de l'Union, Saint Jean, France

BARBARA PICLET LEGRÉ, MD
Centre du Pied 13, Marseille, France

JEFFREY E. McALISTER, DPM, AACFAS
Foot and Ankle Surgeon, Orthopedic Surgery, CORE Institute, Phoenix, Arizona

JENNIFER L. MULHERN, DPM, AACFAS
Foot and Ankle Department, Coordinated Health, Bethlehem, Pennsylvania

BENJAMIN D. OVERLEY Jr, DPM, FACFAS
Foot and Ankle Specialist, Division of Orthopedics, Pottstown Medical Specialists, Inc,
Pottstown, Pennsylvania

KYLE S. PETERSON, DPM, AACFAS
Fellowship-Trained Foot and Ankle Surgeon, Suburban Orthopaedics, Bartlett, Illinois

NICOLE M. PROTZMAN, MS
Clinical Education and Research Department, Coordinated Health, Allentown,
Pennsylvania

DAVID REDFERN, FRCS(Tr&Orth)
London Foot and Ankle Centre, Hospital of St John and St Elizabeth, London, United
Kingdom

RYAN T. SCOTT, DPM, FACFAS
Attending Physician, Department of Orthopedics, The CORE Institute, Phoenix, Arizona

MATTHEW D. SORENSEN, DPM, FACFAS
Fellowship Trained Surgeon, Attending - Advanced Foot and Ankle Reconstruction
Fellowship, Weil Foot and Ankle Institute, Des Plaines, Illinois

JOEL VERNOIS, MD
Sussex Orthopaedic NHS Treatment Center, West Sussex, United Kingdom

LOWELL WEIL Jr, DPM, FACFAS
President of Weil Foot and Ankle Institute, Fellowship Director, Advanced Foot and Ankle
Reconstruction Fellowship, Weil Foot and Ankle Institute, Des Plaines, Illinois

Contents

> Central metatarsal osteotomy is an effective approach in alleviating pain oriented to the forefoot. The procedures individually are straightforward in the isolated scenario. A working knowledge of the specific and unique pathobiomechanics is imperative when considering surgical intervention for the given pathologic scenario. Treating only the pain focus generally underserves the pathology and does not address the high point of the deformity. The surgeon must be cognizant of the complication potpourri, prepare the patient expectations, and engage a level of proactivity against sequelae to ensure the best possible and most predictable outcome.

> This article describes some of the common techniques used in percutaneous surgery of the forefoot. Techniques such as minimally invasive chevron Akin osteotomy for correction of hallux valgus, first metatarsophalangeal joint cheilectomy, distal minimally invasive metatarsal osteotomies, bunionette correction, and hammertoe correction are described. This article is an introduction to this rapidly developing area of foot and ankle surgery. Less invasive techniques are continually being developed across the whole spectrum of surgical specialties. The surgical ethos of minimizing soft-tissue disruption in the process of achieving surgical objectives remains at the center of this evolution.

> A tailor's bunion or bunionette deformity is a combination of osseous and soft tissue bursitis on the lateral aspect of the fifth metatarsal head. This article discusses 7 corrective measures: medial oblique sliding osteotomy with fixation, medial oblique slide osteotomy–minimal incision procedure without fixation, SERI (simple, effective, rapid, inexpensive) with fixation, chevron with or without fixation, closing, lateral wedge osteotomy at the metatarsal neck or proximal diaphysis, Weil osteotomy, and scarfette. These evidence-based techniques can be used by practitioners for medical management of their patients through evaluation, diagnosis, and prognosis. Complications are also addressed.

We present a discussion on the use of proximal first-ray osteotomies in the surgical treatment for hallux valgus as a valid option compared with first-tarsometatarsal arthrodesis. Recent and historical literature tells us that stability of the first ray is a function of the alignment and reestablishment of retrograde stabilizing forces at the first tarsometatarsal joint. This realignment and stabilization may be accomplished with the use of distal soft tissue and proximal osteotomy procedures.

The authors dedicate this article to describing the clinical work-up and etiology for a cavus foot deformity as well as the surgical decision making for correction. Understanding and proper utilization of osteotomies is paramount in the improvement of cavus foot deformities. Also, the authors share their own experiences with preferred techniques for optimal outcomes.

 Video fixation of the posterior calcaneal arm accompanies this article

Flexible adult acquired flatfoot disorder is commonly treated with the use of osteotomies in the calcaneus and medial column. The combination of these joint-preserving osteotomies with additional soft-tissue procedures allows realignment of the hindfoot with the goal of preventing further deformity or degenerative joint disease. A thorough understanding of each patient's condition allows the surgeon to match the correct osteotomy to the clinical indication, while also successfully executing the planned surgery.

Patients with diabetic neuropathy that develop unstable Charcot neuroarthropathy not only have an autoimmune disease that prolongs the healing process, they also often have an inability to maintain a non-weight bearing status. Charcot neuroarthropathy is often devastating to the structure and stability of the foot and ankle. This disease may require permanent bracing, reconstructive surgical stabilization, and in some cases lower leg amputation. Successful management of Charcot neuroarthropathy requires diligence and surveillance by physician and patient alike.

A minimally invasive surgical approach has been developed for hindfoot as well as forefoot procedures. Percutaneous techniques have been evolving for more than 20 years. Many conventional surgical techniques can be performed percutaneously after training. Percutaneous surgical techniques require knowledge specific to each procedure (eg, percutaneous Zadek osteotomy or percutaneous medial heel shift). In the treatment and correction of the hindfoot pathology the surgeon now has percutaneous options including medial or lateral heel shift, Zadek osteotomy, and exostectomy with/without arthroscopy.

CLINICS IN PODIATRIC MEDICINE AND SURGERY

FORTHCOMING ISSUES

October 2015
Secondary Procedures in Total Ankle Replacement
Thomas S. Roukis, *Editor*

January 2016
Tendon Repairs and Transfers for the Foot & Ankle
Christopher L. Reeves, *Editor*

April 2016
Current Update on Foot and Ankle Arthroscopy
Sean T. Grambart, *Editor*

RECENT ISSUES

April 2015
Sports Related Foot & Ankle Injuries
Paul R. Langer, *Editor*

January 2015
Current Update on Orthobiologics in Foot and Ankle Surgery
Barry I. Rosenblum, *Editor*

October 2014
Lower Extremity Complex Trauma and Complications
John J. Stapleton, *Editor*

July 2014
Adult Acquired Flatfoot Deformity
Alan R. Catanzariti and
Robert W. Mendicino, *Editors*

RELATED INTEREST

Foot and Ankle Clinics, March 2015 (Vol. 20, Issue 1)
Arthroscopy and Endoscopy
Rebecca A. Cerrato, *Editor*
Available at: http://www.foot.theclinics.com/

THE CLINICS ARE AVAILABLE ONLINE!
Access your subscription at:
www.theclinics.com

Foreword

Foot and Ankle Osteotomies

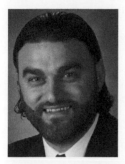

Thomas Zgonis, DPM, FACFAS
Consulting Editor

This issue of *Clinics in Podiatric Medicine and Surgery* is focused on correctional foot and ankle osteotomies collaborated by experienced national and international surgeons. Various topics include metatarsal osteotomies, flatfoot and cavus foot correctional osteotomies, as well as percutaneous and minimal invasive surgery of the forefoot and hindfoot. Further complex foot and ankle deformities are also well covered by contributions on supramalleolar osteotomies and osteotomies for Charcot foot and ankle neuroathropathy.

Our guest editor, Dr Hyer, and invited authors have presented an outstanding scientific work dealing with correctional osteotomies of the foot and ankle. The importance of identifying the origin of deformity along with a thorough clinical, laboratory, radiographic, and medical imaging testing is emphasized throughout this issue. Equal attention is given to the technological advances and fixation methods for the foot and ankle osteotomies. Finally, I hope that this issue by our distinguished national and international authors is helpful when dealing with deformities of the foot and ankle. I would also like to thank the guest editor and all of our contributors and readers for their continuous support in *Clinics in Podiatric Medicine and Surgery*.

Thomas Zgonis, DPM, FACFAS
Division of Podiatric Medicine and Surgery
Department of Orthopedics
University of Texas Health Science Center San Antonio
7703 Floyd Curl Drive–MSC 7776
San Antonio, TX 78229, USA

E-mail address:
zgonis@uthscsa.edu

Clin Podiatr Med Surg 32 (2015) xi
http://dx.doi.org/10.1016/j.cpm.2015.04.002   **podiatric.theclinics.com**
0891-8422/15/$ – see front matter © 2015 Published by Elsevier Inc.

Preface

A Fresh Look at Foot and Ankle Osteotomies

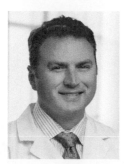

Christopher F. Hyer, DPM, MS, FACFAS
Editor

It is with great pleasure that I present to you an issue dedicated to Foot and Ankle Osteotomies. Corrective osteotomies are commonly used in foot and ankle reconstruction and continue to evolve with time, technologic advances, and enhanced surgeon skill. In this dedicated issue, we have secured some of the best and brightest surgeons from around the world to help update us on the utility of corrective osteotomies and highlight some of the latest techniques in evolution.

I hope you will be as pleased as I am in reading these articles that are laced with both historical review but, more importantly, up-to-date understanding and surgical pearls from some of the very "masters" who have developed these techniques. Our authors are at the forefront on the advances in foot and ankle research and education. In fact, almost every author is either fellowship trained, a fellowship director, or involved in surgeon education and training.

This issue also has the benefit of the presentation of a combined American and European experience as the foot and ankle specialty truly has become worldwide. We can all learn so much from each other, and the different perspectives and experiences presented are a breath of fresh air. In addition, the role of minimally invasive surgery has had a huge resurgence, but only with a thorough and thoughtful development of education, training, and skill set. I expect you will be as excited to read these techniques as I have been. Please enjoy.

Christopher F. Hyer, DPM, MS, FACFAS
Orthopedic Foot & Ankle Center
Westerville Medical Campus
300 Polaris Parkway, Suite 2000
Westerville, OH 43082, USA

E-mail address:
ofacresearch@gmail.com

Clin Podiatr Med Surg 32 (2015) xiii
http://dx.doi.org/10.1016/j.cpm.2015.04.001
0891-8422/15/$ – see front matter © 2015 Published by Elsevier Inc.

podiatric.theclinics.com

Lesser Metatarsal Osteotomy

Matthew D. Sorensen, DPM, FACFAS*, Lowell Weil Jr, DPM, FACFAS

KEYWORDS

- Lesser metatarsal • Weil osteotomy • Plantar plate • Floating toe • Hypermobility

KEY POINTS

- Central metatarsal osteotomy is an effective approach in alleviating pain oriented to the forefoot.
- The procedures individually are straightforward in the isolated scenario.
- A working knowledge of the specific and unique pathobiomechanics is imperative when considering surgical intervention for the given pathologic scenario.
- The surgeon must be cognizant of the complication potpourri, prepare the patient expectations, and engage a level of proactivity against sequelae to ensure the best possible and most predictable outcome.

INTRODUCTION

It is well established that there is no more potentially frustrating pathologic disorder of the foot than that of the lesser metatarsal, particularly when paired with a contracted hammer toe deformity. Adding to the difficult nature of lesser metatarsal pain and hammer toe deformity is the lack of predictability of conservative and surgical intervention. There remains little in the way of blinded, controlled, outcome-driven study to help guide the surgeon's direction of care for patients with the lesser metatarsal malady.

Secondary to the known deficit of predictable treatment options, emphasis must be directed toward knowledge of the pathomechanics contributing to the specific patient complaint. It is well understood that lesser metatarsal pathology can arise from a plethora of biomechanical, genetic, traumatic, and progressive pathologies.[1–19] To give patients the most predictable result with improvement in symptoms, each surgeon must engage a working knowledge of the contributing local

Disclosures: Dr Sorensen – Consultant and Design Surgeon for Stryker Orthopedics and Treace Medical; Dr Weil – Consultant/Design Surgeon for Arthrex and Consultant/Design Surgeon for Treace Medical.
Weil Foot & Ankle Institute, Golf River Professional Building, 1455 East Golf Road, Des Plaines, IL 60016, USA
* Corresponding author.
E-mail address: mdsoren34@gmail.com

and global factors. Treating the obvious problem singularly at the toe or treating only radiographic findings has little place in metatarsalgia and hammer toe corrective intervention. External and more proximal pathology must be considered as well as that which is directly apparent. Treatment of the high point of the deformity is as important in this context as any other treatable pathology; otherwise, one faces subpar predictability and high rates of recurrent pain or concomitant pathology such as the floating toe.

This article addresses lesser metatarsal pathology from the surgical perspective of osteotomy. The importance of concomitant soft-tissue or bony pathology that must be accounted for when considering directed treatment is also discussed. It is accepted that the learning curve for lesser metatarsal procedures, technically, is shallow. The difficulty is associated with the intrinsic pathology, both of bone and soft tissue, and the decision-making threshold in treating concomitant pathology. Unfortunately, there is no standardized protocol in this regard. Subsequently, surgeon expertise, experience, and the art of medicine come at a premium in directing predictable outcomes therein.

CLINICAL EVALUATION

Typical presentation includes specific complaint of lesser metatarsal pain. Evaluation includes isolation of the specific locale of pain. Depending on the pathology, the nidus of pain varies. It is important to assess the history of presentation, including any history of trauma. Insidious onset usually arises secondary to gradual biomechanical developmental deformity and subsequent overload to the lesser metatarsals.

Once the pain locale is isolated, it is important to evaluate the intrinsic high point of deformity. In posttraumatic scenarios, generally the lesser metatarsal pain is secondary to malhealing in the sagittal or transverse plane of a fracture pattern, secondary to direct insult to soft-tissue/capsular structures, or a combination of both.

In the nontraumatic presentation, pain is usually secondary to functional biomechanical fault. This condition can be congenital, occurring in younger age groups, such as brachymetatarsia or short first ray (**Fig. 1**). In addition, lesser metatarsal pain can be seen in populations in which abnormal mechanics have contributed to break down over many years, with sudden pain onset that makes little sense to the patient. The "straw that breaks the camel's back" adage is appropriate here. A global biomechanical evaluation is of utmost importance in such cases. An isolated approach or one of tunnel vision, focusing only on the anatomic pain site, leads to less-than-

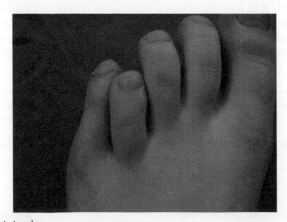

Fig. 1. Brachymetatarsia.

satisfactory results and high rates of failure. Biomechanical components such as medial column hypermobility, ankle equinus, concomitant pes plano valgus foot type, and forefoot- or hindfoot-driven cavus deformity are all entities that can contribute to the incidence of lesser metatarsal pathology and pain. **Fig. 2** is an example of significantly undercorrected flatfoot reconstruction, with subsequent sagittal plane collapse of the medial column and first ray elevation with significant lesser metatarsal overload. Such a situation should not be treated with an isolated approach. Although major reconstruction is not ubiquitously indicated, **Fig. 3** shows appropriate surgical correction of the lesser metatarsal overload among other pathology in this case.

A third entity that can contribute to lesser metatarsal difficulty is that of iatrogenically induced lesser metatarsal pathology. The most common iatrogenic contribution is likely that of previous bunionectomy in which medial column hypermobility or overload mechanics are underaddressed and second ray insufficiency fracture can be experienced (**Fig. 4**). Bunionectomies in which excessive first ray shortening has occurred can also induce a lack of appropriate load at the first metatarsophalangeal joint (MTPJ). Whenever previous surgical care is a part of the patient history, careful attention should be paid to potential iatrogenic pathomechanics. When the deficit is identified, one must take care, in full understanding, of the deficit and address the mechanics intrinsic to and in accord with the lesser metatarsal pain. Ignoring iatrogenic lesser metatarsal pain causes a chasing-of-the-tail–type scenario for the patient and surgeon and can easily be avoided.

RADIOGRAPHIC ANALYSIS

Radiographic evaluation remains the gold standard for static evaluation of metatarsal length and alignment in the context of surrounding osseous structures (**Fig. 5**). However, radiographs are only a component to the evaluation, and one cannot rely solely on these findings. Gait pattern pathologies, particularly at the midstance and toe-off phases of gait, are a dynamic process with functional implications, and therefore, radiographs must be evaluated in this context. Findings on radiographs of static stance weight bearing depend on the positions of the foot and the x-ray beam. Minor changes in either entity can have significant implication in the resultant radiographic representation of the structural osseous status throughout the forefoot and metatarsal parabola therein.

In addition, there is no truly defined normal in the context of the transverse plane distal metatarsal parabola.[17,20] Proposals have been introduced with indication for

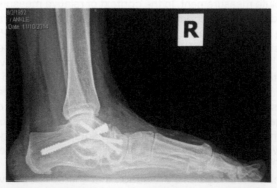

Fig. 2. First ray elevation secondary to hindfoot malposition and sagittal plane collapse.

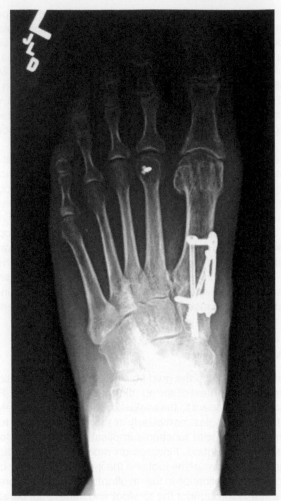

Fig. 3. First tarsometatarsal fusion performed to stabilize medial column hypermobility in a case of lesser metatarsal overload.

relative and absolute measurement. In the context of relative measurement, a gradual taper is expected to progress from the second to the fifth metatarsal, with the first metatarsal being somewhat shorter than the second (2>1 = 3>4>5). In contrast, it has been suggested that the first and second metatarsals should be of equal length (1 = 2>3>4>5).[21–26] Tangential measurements can be drawn to evaluate the taper of the lesser metatarsals (**Fig. 6**).[27] The noted limitation intrinsic to these measurements, however, is the assumption that the 2 reference points (distal aspects of the 2 lesser metatarsals) are normal. Absolute measurements can be derived from the variation off tangential lines and also through the classic system proposed by Hardy and Clapham[28] in 1951 (**Fig. 6**). These measurements give the surgeon a quantified goal for transverse plane surgical correction that can be approximated intraoperatively.[29]

A final component of radiographic evaluation that should not be overlooked in scenarios of lesser metatarsal pain is that of cortical hypertrophy. Secondary to Wolff's

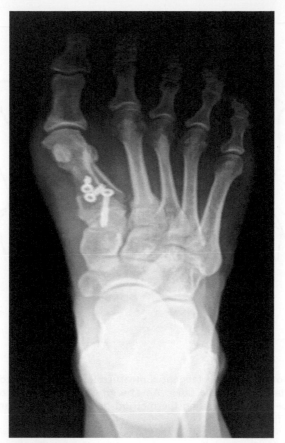

Fig. 4. Second metatarsal insufficiency fracture shown secondary to iatrogenically induced first ray insufficiency after attempted bunionectomy.

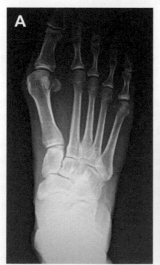

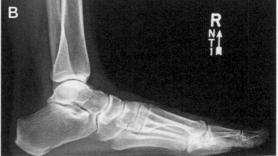

Fig. 5. Classic anteroposterior (*A*) and lateral (*B*) foot radiographs necessary for the first-line hallux valgus evaluation.

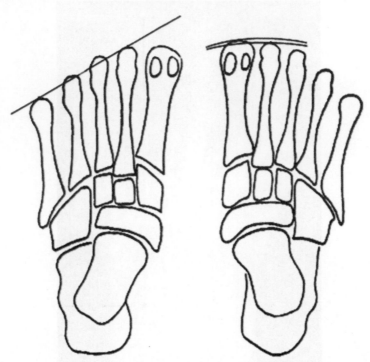

Fig. 6. The left foot shows how a tangential measurement can be used to quantify the expected lesser metatarsal parabola taper. An absolute measurement between 2 adjacent metatarsals can be determined using the method described first by Hardy and Clapham (*right foot* in the figure).

law, the body inherently deposits a more robust level of calcification to areas that are under increased stress. When the lesser metatarsal middiaphyseal shafts, particularly that of the second ray, are hypertrophied compared with what would be expected, this may be a signal that significant overload is occurring secondary to insufficiency or deficit in full weight bearing at the first ray.

MRI or computed tomographic advanced imaging is generally not necessary unless there is concern over potential avascular necrosis, Freiberg infraction, or concern over healing of a previous fracture (**Fig. 7**). In addition, when there is concern with regard to concomitant soft-tissue pathology such as a plantar plate tear, high-resolution MRI can aid in preoperative evaluation, as well as to educate the patient on the severity of the pathology involved with the pain. Threshold to order such a study should be low in these circumstances so as not to set the patient up for inadvertent failure.

Ultrasonic evaluation is a fourth modality that can significantly aid in evaluation of soft-tissue pathology in and around the forefoot. Impact on the patient is low when engaging this modality, and patients appreciate visualizing the pathology with their own eyes; however, the practitioner must have an appropriate level of comfort with their diagnostic skill in using ultrasonography if one is relying on this modality alone.

CONSERVATIVE CARE

It is important to mention conservative care in the treatment regimen, although it is not the scope of this article. Often, care measures such as immobilization, change in shoe gear, accommodative padding, anti-inflammatories, functional orthoses, strapping of

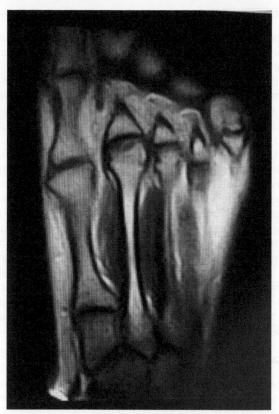

Fig. 7. Advanced MRI showing significant second metatarsal head Freiberg infraction.

toes, and formal physical therapy can help substantially. The goal with these treatment modalities is aimed reduction of intra-articular synovitis or other soft-tissue inflammatory change through accommodation of structural or functional deformity inherent to the pathology.[30–35] Despite the relative paucity of peer-reviewed material directing and guiding the surgeon in the benefit of conservative intervention, arthrocentesis using local anesthetic can be used to give temporary relief and aid in diagnosis with the secondary benefit of giving patients a real-time picture of what the joint might feel like when ultimately healed. The authors do not routinely use intra-articular injection of corticosteroid, whether short acting or long acting. Although this modality does predictably provide pain relief, it is a finite intervention and has significant potential of further attenuating already damaged capsular structures; this can cause the deformity to prematurely progress and ultimately increase the level of difficulty if surgical intervention becomes necessary in the future.

Other than in the posttraumatic population, it is understood and should be communicated to patients that these treatment entities will not fix the problem and only accommodate the symptoms, which many times is enough to buy patients time. Depending on patient expectations for activity, or in those who are poor surgical candidates, conservative entities can be a long-term option.

Ultimately, however, even with good conservative care, the pathology is progressive and generally necessitates a definitive approach. Again, it is incumbent on the physician to communicate appropriate patient perspective in this regard.

LESSER METATARSAL VASCULAR ANATOMY

The vascular supply to the central metatarsals has been well established in several anatomic studies.[36–38] The arcuate artery, arising from the dorsalis pedis artery, sends dorsal metatarsal arteries through the intermetatarsal spaces over the dorsal interosseous muscles that produce a well-defined dorsal capsular network to each of the MTPJs. The dorsal capsular branches anastomose with each other and with the plantar capsular vessels to form a dense periarticular network that produces 1 of 2 fine vessels that supply the metatarsal head at the level of the extra-articular dorsal synovial fold and collateral ligament attachments. The planar arch, arising from the lateral plantar artery division of the posterior tibial artery, sends plantar metatarsal arteries through the intermetatarsal spaces between the plantar interosseous muscles and the oblique head of the adductor hallucis muscle. These vessels produce a well-defined and robust branch that divides into 2 clearly defined terminal branches at the level of the plantar metatarsal metaphyseal-diaphyseal junction and proximal attachment of the plantar plate. One branch supplies the plantar capsular structures including the plantar plate and anastomoses with the dorsal capsular branches, and the other supplies the metatarsal head itself.[36–38] The nutrient artery and periosteal vessels are also important and supply the metaphyseal and cortical components of the metatarsal, respectively.[36,38] However, because this article focuses on central metatarsal head-neck osteotomies, any osteotomy at this level should limit soft-tissue dissection through the interspaces, about the capsule and periosteal structures, and spare the plantar metaphyseal-diaphyseal junction.[15]

CENTRAL METATARSAL OSTEOTOMIES

Numerous osteotomies have been described in the literature toward the aim of relieving plantar lesser metatarsal pain. Most are in effort to shorten the metatarsal or elevate the head or both while simultaneously decompressing the metatarsal-phalangeal joint. Central or proximal metatarsal osteotomies historically have been reserved for scenarios in which there is lack of deformity at the MTPJ itself but persistent plantar metatarsal pain is present. This situation is more commonly seen in the posttraumatic patient profile, whereby there is no need to address capsular deformity. Midshaft or proximal osteotomies include the telescoping osteotomy, sagittal scarf-type osteotomy, or variations on a sagittal chevron osteotomy (**Fig. 8**). In addition, Barouk[25] has published on a proximal dorsal wedge-type osteotomy.

The midshaft osteotomy is also indicated in brachymetatarsia, in which case significant increase in length is required. External fixation concomitant with corticotomy is often used with periods of off-loading. A pearl to add when performing callus distraction for brachymetatarsia is to pin the toe with a smooth Kirschner wire across the MTPJ so as to prevent contracture at the distal joints during the distraction period. The pin should be kept in place long enough after distraction to allow the soft-tissues to calm down and decrease the incidence of toe contracture.[1,7,11,39–46]

A well-known concern with proximal or midshaft osteotomies is the inherent instability of such osteotomies given their location and substantial cantilever force loads that translate through this portion of the foot with weight bearing. Historically, midshaft osteotomy has required significant periods of off-loading postoperation, with inherent increased risks. New-generation locked plating technology that is anatomy specific may decrease the time to weight bearing secondary to the increased level of rigidity and use external fixation principles internally and make these midshaft procedures

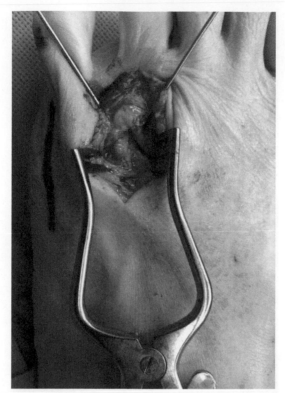

Fig. 8. Clinical picture illustrating sagittal chevron osteotomy.

more palatable for patients and surgeons (**Fig. 9**). Short- and long-term studies, however, are lacking in reference to actual decrease in off-loading time when using the capacities of locked plates.

The inherent tenuous blood supply, as discussed previously, at the single nutrient artery of the central metatarsals can lead to difficulty with healing even with extended periods of off-loading. Minimally invasive approaches with special attention on soft-tissue handling have been described with effort to decrease the incidence of vascular embarrassment and subsequent healing sequelae.[47] Application of appropriate fixation can prove difficult in the minimally invasive scenario, and so cost-benefit must be weighed when using minimally invasive approaches.

Weil Osteotomy

The most popularized lesser metatarsal osteotomy aimed at lesser metatarsal pathology in recent years is the Weil osteotomy. The reproducibility, inherent stability, robust blood supply at the metatarsal head, ease of execution in addition to effectiveness of the procedure, and subsequent patient satisfaction are some of the important indications for its popularity. In addition, the osteotomy can be easily modified to address triplanar deformity at the MTPJ, furthering the adaptability of its application in lesser metatarsal pathology.

The surgical technique is straight forward. Incision is directed over the dorsal aspect the lesser MTPJ. The authors prefer a straight dorsal incision placement that can easily be extended onto the distal digit when necessary for concomitant procedures.

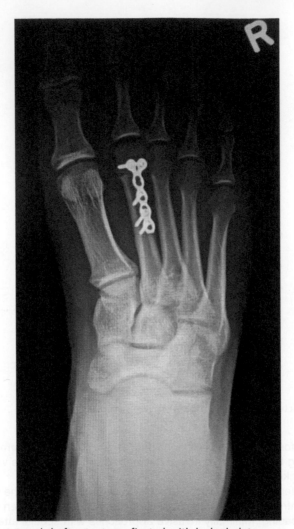

Fig. 9. Lesser metatarsal shaft osteotomy fixated with locked plate.

Appropriate internal and external splinting (**Fig. 10**) may be necessary postoperatively to decrease dorsal scar contracture and floating toe sequelae. Once deep dissection has commenced, attention is directed either medial or lateral to the extensor tendon and longitudinal capsulotomy is performed. The authors recommend the capsulotomy be performed on the laterality where most significant pathologic contracture is identified so as to naturally relax the contracted capsular tissues. Once capsulotomy has been performed, the medial and lateral collateral ligaments can be released to expose the metatarsal head. Next, the distal digit is plantarflexed to further expose the metatarsal head (**Fig. 11**). A sagittal saw is then obtained and used to perform the osteotomy. The osteotomy is intra-articular, beginning at the dorsal extent of the articular cartilage and made parallel to the functional weight-bearing surface. Once the osteotomy is made through the proximal-plantar cortex a small elevator may be necessary to release the proximal periosteum through the osteotomy. The capital fragment is then transposed proximally and can be manipulated in the transverse plane where

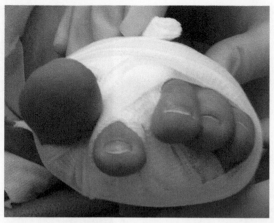

Fig. 10. Postoperative bandaging serving as an external splint allowing soft-tissue consolidation in the immediate healing phase.

necessary to address deformity in this plane. Many times, on punching through the proximal extent of the osteotomy, the capital fragment finds its own level; however, care should be taken to ensure that the metatarsal is not overshortened, inducing a potential floating toe. On finding the appropriate level of the capital fragment, it is fixated using 1 or 2 points of fixation (**Fig. 12**). The authors prefer engaging a 2.0-mm twist-off screw; however, any combination of fixation techniques may be used. Once fixation has commenced, the remaining dorsal shelf should be excised using a bone rongeur to allow appropriate dorsiflexion of the toe on the metatarsal.

Concomitant soft-tissue or further distal digital work can then be performed as necessary. Generally, the authors do not actively close the deep capsule, so as to prevent potential overzealous scar and subsequent contracture. The toe is splinted in slight plantarflexory attitude to allow the soft tissue to heal appropriately.

When performed in an isolated fashion, the authors allow immediate WBAT (weight bearing as tolerated) in a postoperative shoe with gradual transition to shoes. The toe

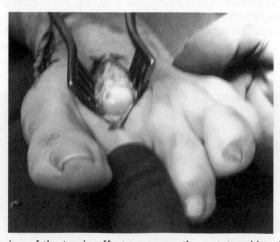

Fig. 11. Plantarflexion of the toe in effort to expose the metatarsal head for osteotomy.

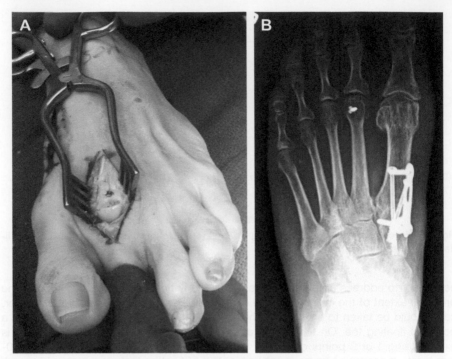

Fig. 12. Fixation used in the Weil osteotomy clinical (*A*) and radiographic (*B*).

is splinted or strapped on skin healing. Ultimately, concomitant procedures often dictate the postoperative course to weight bearing and rehabilitation.

FLOATING TOE

The most common or most complained complication of the Weil osteotomy is the floating toe seen in conjunction with a lesser digit proximal interphalangeal joint (PIPJ) fusion; this is defined as the incapacity of the toe to appropriately purchase the weight-bearing surface during midstance (**Fig. 13**). Formation of a hammer toe, whereby deformity includes sagittal plane contracture or transverse plane deviation, also includes a significant retrograde contracture force on the metatarsal head pushing it plantarward on the normal parabola.[48] In these scenarios, the plantar plate is likely to have significant attenuation or partial rupture, and this is where evaluation

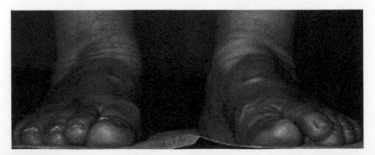

Fig. 13. Floating toe example noted to the left second digit.

of the high point of the deformity is imperative. If the underlying pathology creating the lesser metatarsal pain is not addressed, complications are inevitable.[15,17,21,49]

Floating toe is widely recognized as a common sequel of the Weil osteotomy. The literature is full of articles indicating the rate of floating toe sequelae from the Weil osteotomy in particular. Rates ranging from 15% to 50% have been reported.[2,4,8,11]

Several postulations as to the formation of the floating toe have been presented. One theory points to the significant relaxation of the surrounding tissues that occurs with shortening of the metatarsal head. It is thought that when the soft tissues, and particularly the extensor and most importantly the flexor tendons, relax, they lose their power on the toe and it begins to migrate accordingly secondary to excess slack in the tendons. Thus, it is important to consider maintaining physiologic tension to the surrounding soft tissues.[29] In addition, the plantar plate likely takes on a change in loading pattern, further driving sagittal plane difficulty.

A second theory concerning the development of a floating toe was presented by Trnka and colleagues,[7] who studied the floating toe pathology specifically via performing the osteotomy both on sawbones and cadaveric specimen. He found it difficult to actually perform the osteotomy parallel to the weight-bearing surface, and in many instances the bone cut was placed more vertically. The sequelae therein include an unintentional depression of the capital fragment on proximal translation. Subsequently, they described a translation of the center of rotation on the long axis of the interosseous muscles and the resultant kinematics on the toe. Instead of having the normal impact on toe flexion, they became dorsally oriented on the metatarsal head and therefore became dorsiflexors at the digit rather than transverse plane stability.[7,8]

Although floating toe is a well-accepted risk of metatarsal head decompression osteotomy, there are ways to prevent the frustrating sequelae. There is room for the use of dorsal structure lengthening, such as an extensor tendon lengthening. Dorsal lengthening alone, however, is not advised, as this does not address the plantar laxity within the plantar plate or flexor tendons and thus only weakens the toe without any significant effect in preventing migration of the toe into dorsiflexion.

When a floating toe is to be avoided, any dorsal work must be concomitant to plantar reefing at the plantar plate or via a flexor tendon transfer in conjunction with a PIPJ fusion. Although it is not the scope of this article to specifically address these 2 plantar approaches, they are reliable options in maintaining a plantarflexed posture of the proximal phalanx on the metatarsal head.

A second option, which has room for controversy, is pinning the toe into place. The concept of pinning the toe across the MTPJ is an effort to place the toe in its corrected position in the sagittal and transverse planes, with the goal of allowing the soft-tissue structures to scar in around the pinned toe. The thought, therefore, is that once the pin is pulled at 4 to 6 weeks, the scarred-in soft-tissue structures will maintain appropriate alignment of position. Unfortunately, on pulling the pin, it is not uncommon to see the toe migrate dorsally. Thus, reliance on the pin is generally underserving of the pathology, and focus must remain on repair of the plantar structures or flexor transfer.

Additional points of contention regarding cross-MTPJ pinning include potential displacement of the metatarsal osteotomy performed on driving the pin into the head. This displacement creates a more complicated fixation dilemma for the osteotomy and certainly increases tourniquet time. Iatrogenic arthrosis may be induced if the pin is not placed in the desired location on the metatarsal on the first try. Repeated attempts at placement of the pin increase damage to the articular surface. Sausage digit is also a known potential consequence of pinning of the toes, secondary to vascular embarrassment from overextension of the toe on the pin. Lastly, pin breakage can occur within the toe or within the joint secondary to lack of awareness by the patient.

SUMMARY

Central metatarsal osteotomy is an effective approach in alleviating pain oriented to the forefoot. The procedures individually are straightforward in the isolated scenario. A working knowledge of the specific and unique pathobiomechanics is imperative when considering surgical intervention for the given pathologic scenario. Treating only the pain focus generally underserves the pathology and does not address the high point of the deformity. Contributing biomechanical drivers other than that readily apparent must be considered and treated accordingly. In addition, lesser metatarsal osteotomy does not come without potential complication. The surgeon must be cognizant of the complication potpourri, prepare the patient expectations, and engage a level of proactivity against sequelae to ensure the best possible and most predictable outcome.

REFERENCES

1. Trnka HJ, Mühlbauer M, Zettl R, et al. Comparison of the results of the Weil and Helal osteotomies for the treatment of metatarsalgia secondary to dislocation of the lesser metatarsophalangeal joint. Foot Ankle Int 1999;20:72–9.
2. O'Kane C, Kilmartin TE. The surgical management of central metatarsalgia. Foot Ankle Int 2002;23(5):415–9.
3. Cheng YM, Lin SY, Wu CK. Oblique sliding metatarsal osteotomy for pressure metatarsalgia. Gaoxiong Yi Xue Ke Xue Za Zhi 1992;8(8):403–11.
4. Beech I, Rees S, Tagoe M. A retrospective review of the Weil metatarsalosteotomy for lesser metatarsal deformities: an intermediate follow-up analysis. J Foot Ankle Surg 2005;44(5):358–64.
5. Kennedy JG, Deland JT. Resolution of metatarsalgia following oblique osteotomy. Clin Orthop Relat Res 2006;453:309–13.
6. Okuda R, Kinoshita M, Morikawa J, et al. Proximal metatarsalosteotomy: relation between 1- to greater than 3-years results. Clin Orthop Relat Res 2005;435: 191–6.
7. Trnka HJ, Nyska M, Parks BG, et al. Dorsiflexion contracture after the Weil osteotomy: results of cadaver study and three-dimensional analysis. Foot Ankle Int 2001;22(1):47–50.
8. Migues A, Slullitel G, Bilbao F, et al. Floating-toe deformity as a complication of the Weil osteotomy. Foot Ankle Int 2004;25(9):609–13.
9. Schwartz N, Williams JE Jr, Marcinko DE. Double oblique lesser metatarsal osteotomy. J Am Podiatry Assoc 1983;73(4):218–20.
10. Lauf E, Weinraub GM. Asymmetric "V" osteotomy: a predictable surgical approach for chronic central metatarsalgia. J Foot Ankle Surg 1996;35(6):550–9.
11. Vandeputte G, Dereymaeker G, Steenwerckx A, et al. The Weil osteotomy of the lesser metatarsals: a clinical and pedobarographic follow-up study. Foot Ankle Int 2000;21(5):370–4.
12. Idusuyi OB, Kitaoka HB, Patzer GL. Oblique metatarsal osteotomy for intractable plantar keratosis: 10-year follow-up. Foot Ankle Int 1998;19(6):351–5.
13. Hatcher RM, Gollier WL, Weil LS. Intractable plantar keratoses: a review of surgical corrections. J Am Podiatr Med Assoc 1978;68:377–86.
14. Pontious J, Lane GD, Moritz JC, et al. Lesser metatarsal V-osteotomy for chronic intractable plantar keratosis. Retrospective analysis of 40 procedures. J Am Podiatr Med Assoc 1998;88(7):323–31.
15. Roukis TS. Central metatarsal head-neck osteotomies: indications and operative techniques. Clin Podiatr Med Surg 2005;22(2):197–222.

16. Jimenez AL, Fishco WD. Part 3: central metatarsals. In: Banks AS, Downey MS, Martin DE, et al, editors. McGlamry's comprehensive textbook of foot and ankle surgery. Philadelphia: Lippincott, Williams and Wilkins; 2001. p. 322–38.
17. Barouk LS. Weil's metatarsal osteotomy in the treatment of metatarsalgia. Orthopade 1996;25(4):338–44.
18. Dockery GL. Evaluation and treatment of metatarsalgia and keratotic disorders. In: Myerson MS, editor. Foot and ankle disorders. Philadelphia: W.B. Saunders Company; 2000. p. 359–78.
19. Khalafi A, Landsman AS, Lautenschlager EP, et al. Plantar forefoot changes after second metatarsal neck osteotomy. Foot Ankle Int 2005;26(7):550–5.
20. Griffin NL, Richmond BG. Cross-sectional geometry of the human forefoot. Bone 2005;37(2):253–6.
21. Viladot A. Metatarsalgia due to biomechanical alterations of the forefoot. Orthop Clin North Am 1973;4(1):165–78.
22. Dominguez G, Munuera PV, Lafuente G. Relative metatarsal protrusion in the adult: a preliminary study. J Am Podiatr Med Assoc 2006;96(3):238–44.
23. Sanner WH. Foot segmental relationships and bone morphology. In: Christman RA, editor. Foot and ankle radiology. St Louis (MO): Churchill Livingstone; 2003. p. 272–302.
24. Bojsen-Møller F. Normal and pathologic anatomy of metatarsals. Orthopade 1982;11(4):148–53.
25. Barouk LS. Metatarsalgia: metatarsal excess of length in dorso-plantar x-ray view in standing position. In: Barouk LS, editor. Forefoot reconstruction. Paris: Springer-Verlag; 2003. p. 214–6.
26. Maestro M, Besse JL, Ragusa M, et al. Forefoot morphotype study and planning method for forefoot osteotomy. Foot Ankle Clin 2003;8(4):695–710.
27. Valley BA, Reese HW. Guidelines for reconstructing the metatarsal parabola with the shortening osteotomy. J Am Podiatr Med Assoc 1991;81(8):406–13.
28. Hardy RH, Clapham JC. Observations on hallux valgus based on a controlled series. J Bone Joint Surg Br 1951;33-B:376–91.
29. Derner R, Meyr AJ. Complications and salvage of elective central metatarsal osteotomies. Clin Podiatr Med Surg 2009;26:23–35.
30. Scranton PE Jr. Metatarsalgia: a clinical review of diagnosis and management. Foot Ankle 1981;1(4):229–34.
31. Trepal MJ, Harkless LB, Jules KT, et al. Central metatarsalgia. Preferred practice guideline. Park Ridge (IL): American College of Foot and Ankle Surgeons; 1998. p. 2–35.
32. Holmes GB, Timmerman L. A quantitative assessment of the effect of metatarsal pads of plantar pressures. Foot Ankle 1990;11(3):141–5.
33. Chang AH, Abu-Faraj ZU, Harris GF, et al. Multistep measurement of plantar pressure alterations using metatarsal pads. Foot Ankle Int 1994;15(12):654–60.
34. Poon C, Love B. Efficacy of foot orthotics for metatarsalgia. Foot 1997;7(4):202–4.
35. Postema K, Burn PE, Zande ME, et al. Primary metatarsalgia: influence of a custom moulded insole and a rockerbar on plantar pressure. Prosthet Orthot Int 1998;22(1):35–44.
36. Jaworek TE. Intrinsic vascular alterations within osseous tissue of the lesser metatarsals. Arch Podiatr Med Foot Surg 1978;5(2):9–22.
37. Leemrijse T, Valtin B, Oberlin C. Vascularization of the heads of the three central metatarsals: an anatomical study, its application and considerations with respect to horizontal osteotomies at the neck of the metatarsals. Foot Ankle Surg 1998;4: 57–62.

38. Petersen WJ, Lankes JM, Paulsen F, et al. The arterial supply of the lesser metatarsal heads: a vascular injection study in human cadavers. Foot Ankle Int 2002; 23(6):491–5.
39. Barouk LS. The Weil metatarsal osteotomy. In: Forefoot reconstruction. Paris: Springer-Verlag; 2003. p. 109–32.
40. Weil LS Sr. Weil head-neck oblique osteotomy: technique and fixation. Presented at Techniques of Osteotomies of the Forefoot. Bordeaux (France), October 20–22, 1994.
41. Rochwerger A, Launay F, Piclet B, et al. Static instability and dislocation of the second metatarsophalangeal joint: comparative analysis of two different therapeutic modalities. Rev Chir Orthop Reparatrice Appar Mot 1998;84(5):433–9.
42. Maceira E, Fariñas F, Tena J, et al. Large metatarsal shortenings and postoperative stiffness. Foot Ankle Int 1999;20(10):677–83.
43. Mqhlbauer M, Trnka HJ, Zembsch A, et al. Short-term outcome of Weil osteotomy in treatment of metatarsalgia. Z Orthop Ihre Grenzgeb 1999;137(5):452–6.
44. Davies MS, Saxby TS. Metatarsal neck osteotomy with rigid internal fixation for the treatment of lesser toe metatarsophalangeal joint pathology. Foot Ankle Int 1999;20(10):630–5.
45. Tollafield DR. An audit of lesser metatarsal osteotomy by capital proximal displacement. [Weil osteotomy] Br J Podiatr 2001;4(1):15–9.
46. Melamed EA, Schon LC, Myerson MS, et al. Two modifications of the Weil osteotomy: analysis on sawbone model. Foot Ankle Int 2002;23(5):400–5.
47. White DL. Minimal incision approach to osteotomies of the lesser metatarsals for treatment of intractable keratosis, metatarsalgia, and tailor's bunion. Clin Podiatr Med Surg 1991;8(1):25–39.
48. Yu GV, Judge MS, Hudson JR, et al. Predislocation syndrome. Progressive subluxation/dislocation of the lesser metarsophalangeal joint. J Am Podiatr Med Assoc 2002;92(4):182–99.
49. Hofstaetter SG, Hofstaetter JG, Petroutsas JA, et al. The Weil osteotomy: a seven-year follow-up. J Bone Joint Surg Br 2005;87(11):1507–11.

Percutaneous Surgery of the Forefoot

David Redfern, FRCS(Tr&Orth)[a],*, Joel Vernois, MD[b], Barbara Piclet Legré, MD[c]

KEYWORDS

- MIS • Percutaneous • Forefoot • Hallux valgus • Hammer • Rigidus

KEY POINTS

- In overview, minimally invasive chevron Akin (MICA) is a chevron-shaped first metatarsal osteotomy and an Akin-type osteotomy of the proximal phalanx (P1) of the hallux.
- These osteotomies are performed percutaneously with a burr under image intensifier guidance and then rigidly internally fixed with screws.
- A percutaneous soft-tissue release may be performed involving division of the lateral sesamoid:phalangeal ligament (lateral head of flexor hallucis brevis distal to the fibular sesamoid).

In foot and ankle surgery, percutaneous techniques were first explored by Morton Polokoff in 1945 and later by Leonard Britton.[1] Wilson[2] and Bosch and colleagues[3] have subsequently also promoted minimally invasive techniques. However, it was probably Stephen Isham[4] who attracted a wider interest from the orthopedic community when he published a modification of the Reverdin osteotomy[5] in 1991. Interest has subsequently grown across Europe. Since the turn of the new millennia further publications have appeared.[6–9] De Prado and colleagues[10] from Spain have also been influential in this field.

MINIMALLY INVASIVE CHEVRON AKIN FOR CORRECTION OF HALLUX VALGUS

There have been more than 130 different operations described for the surgical correction of hallux valgus.[11] The MICA procedure is the first percutaneous technique for correction of hallux valgus to combine percutaneous osteotomies with the benefits of modern rigid internal fixation. This technique was first described by Vernois and Redfern[12–16] in 2011, and other surgeons are also beginning to publish their results with this and similar percutaneous techniques.

[a] London Foot and Ankle Centre, Hospital of St John and St Elizabeth, 60 Grove End Road, London NW8 9NH, UK; [b] Sussex Orthopaedic Treatment Centre, West Sussex, UK; [c] Centre du Pied 13, Marseille, France
* Corresponding author.
E-mail address: david.redfern@springgroup.org

Clin Podiatr Med Surg 32 (2015) 291–332
http://dx.doi.org/10.1016/j.cpm.2015.03.007
0891-8422/15/$ – see front matter © 2015 Elsevier Inc. All rights reserved.

In overview, the MICA procedure is a chevron-shaped first metatarsal osteotomy and an Akin-type osteotomy of the P1 of the hallux. These osteotomies are performed percutaneously with a burr under image intensifier guidance and then rigidly internally fixed with screws. In addition, a percutaneous soft-tissue release may be performed involving division of the lateral sesamoid:phalangeal ligament (lateral head of flexor hallucis brevis distal to the fibular sesamoid).

Indications/Contraindications

In terms of radiologic severity, the MICA procedure is indicated for mild to moderate hallux valgus deformities, but with experience, the surgeon can quite reasonably extend the indications to treat more severe deformities as long as 100% lateral displacement of the metatarsal head is sufficient to correct the intermetatarsal angle.

In addition to the aforementioned indications, patients with hallux valgus with poor soft tissues or a history of keloid scarring can also be a good indication for the MICA technique.

Furthermore, this technique can be useful in the revision situation, as the percutaneous extracapsular technique minimizes further vascular insult (and stiffness). The MICA procedure also involves a plane of screw fixation different from most open osteotomies, and hence, this can also be useful in the revision situation.

The main contraindications are active infection and critical arterial occlusive disease.

Surgical Technique

1. Equipment
   Burrs: 2 × 20-mm Shannon burr, 2 × 12-mm Shannon burr
   Driver: System with ability to control speed and torque (saline irrigation for cooling also preferable). The ability to control both speed and torque is important as the authors recommend use of very low burr speeds (<500 rpm) and high torque (eg, 80 Ncm) to avoid the risk of skin or soft-tissue burns (and also minimize thermal injury to bone)
   Instruments: Beaver blade, percutaneous elevators
   Mini C-arm (rather than large C-arm), as this is both more maneuverable in obtaining anteroposterior (AP) and lateral views and delivers a very low dose of radiation to both patient and surgeon
   Tourniquet: Not required but depends on surgeon preference. If using a tourniquet, then saline cooling of the burr must be used, as the cooling effect of bleeding at the point of burr entry is lost
2. Anesthesia (either general or regional is administered) and intravenous antibiotics as per local guidelines
3. Positioning: The patient is positioned supine with the feet overhanging the end of the operating table (**Fig. 1**). The mini C-arm is positioned to the right of the patient regardless of which foot is being operated on (left side for left-handed surgeon)

Chevron osteotomy

4. The surgeon creates a chevron osteotomy of the distal first metatarsal at the distal diaphyseal metaphyseal junction using a 20-mm Shannon burr.
   A Beaver blade is used to create a skin portal on the dorsomedial aspect of the first metatarsal at the level of the intended osteotomy (**Fig. 2**). A curved elevator is used to create a working space over the dorsal aspect of the metatarsal and free the lateral periosteum, but this should never be used on the plantar aspect

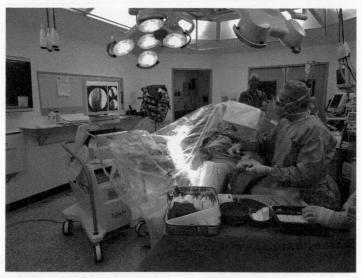

Fig. 1. Theater arrangement for forefoot minimum incision surgery.

of the metatarsal to respect/preserve the blood supply to the metatarsal head. The dorsomedial cutaneous nerve must also be respected in the positioning of the portal and subsequent use of the burr.

A 20-mm Shannon burr is then inserted through the medial cortex of the metatarsal to create the apex of the chevron under image intensifier guidance (see **Fig. 2**). Only when the surgeon is happy with the plane of the apex of the chevron is the burr advanced through the second (lateral) cortex. This step is important, as it dictates the whole plane of the osteotomy.

The 20-mm Shannon burr is 2 mm in diameter and cuts a slot in the bone of 2 to 2.5 mm, which is more than the kerf of an oscillating saw used for open surgery; this must be accounted for in the plane of the chevron osteotomy. To maintain neutral first metatarsal length, the burr should be directed 10° beyond perpendicular to the second metatarsal (distal direction) and 10° in a plantar direction to avoid elevation (**Fig. 3**).

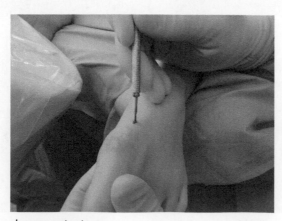

Fig. 2. Incision for chevron osteotomy.

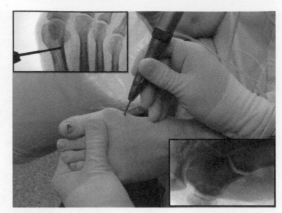

Fig. 3. Chevron osteotomy.

Once happy with the plane of the osteotomy (apex cut), the dorsal and plantar limbs of the chevron are created. The dorsal limb should be perpendicular to the plane of the metatarsal. The plantar limb should be parallel to the floor. The angle of the chevron created is greater than or equal to 90°.

5. Once the osteotomy is completed, the next step is to position the proximal screw guidewire (4-mm screw recommended) in the metatarsal ready to be advanced into the head once the head has been displaced into the desired position (**Fig. 4**). A stab incision is made proximal to the first tarsometatarsal joint through which the guidewire enters the proximal metaphysis right at its base and is advanced obliquely so that it exits the lateral wall of the first metatarsal just proximal to the osteotomy site. The wire should not be advanced any further at this stage; otherwise, it may impede displacement of the osteotomy.

6. To displace the osteotomy, a 2-mm wire or the straight elevator (or other purpose-made instrument) is inserted via the osteotomy portal and into the proximal first metatarsal medullary canal. The head can then be levered laterally. The levering

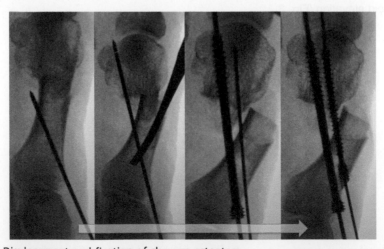

Fig. 4. Displacement and fixation of chevron osteotomy.

instrument pivots on the medial metatarsal wall, and care should be taken not to fracture this in elderly/soft bone.

The levering maneuver involves ensuring that the levering instrument remains positioned over the summit of the bunion. If it slips dorsal, then the metatarsal head fragment is plantar-flexed. If it slips plantar to the bunion, then the head fragment is dorsiflexed. The surgeon must also control for the tendency for the head fragment to rotate (as well as the desired translation) laterally. This rotation can be avoided by applying varus force to the hallux itself during the maneuver (**Fig. 5**).

7. Once the desired displacement of the metatarsal head has been achieved, the position is controlled with the nondominant hand (NDH) while the guidewire (already positioned in readiness in step 5) is advanced into the head. It is then vital to check the displacement and screw position in both AP and lateral planes. If not satisfactory, then the process of displacement and guidewire advancement is repeated. Once satisfactory positioning of the head fragment and the guidewire fixation has been achieved, the wire is measured and an appropriate screw length inserted (diameter of 4 mm recommended for large displacements). Before drilling for screw insertion, it is recommended to advance the guidewire through the foot and place a clip on the distal end. In this way, the surgeon can always recover both ends if it were to break during the cannulated drilling (**Fig. 6**).

8. A second screw is then inserted just distal to the first in the same plane or slightly divergent (3-mm-diameter screw will suffice) to control rotation. This screw does not need to pass through both cortices of the proximal metatarsal fragment. Redfern uses a MICA screw, which has been specifically designed for this method of fixation and maintains circumferential cortical fix when inserted flush to the bone owing to the flanged head design. Traditional flat-ended screws may easily loosen, back out, and subsequently require removal some months later.

9. Once the osteotomy is fixed, the guidewires are removed and the redundant prominent medial wall of the first metatarsal is removed with a wedge burr (inserted through the proximal screw entry portal working from plantar to dorsal so as not to place the dorsomedial nerve at risk of injury) (**Fig. 7**).

10. If the bunion eminence needs reducing, then this can be done with a wedge burr via the osteotomy portal working from inside the bone to outside in a medial direction.

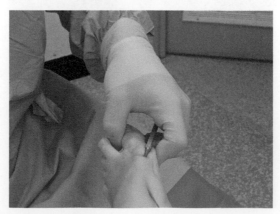

Fig. 5. Correct displacement technique of chevron osteotomy.

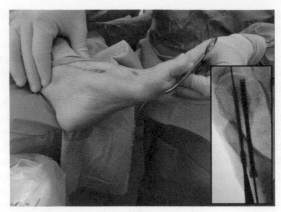

Fig. 6. Fixation technique of chevron osteotomy.

Distal soft-tissue release

11. A distal soft-tissue release is only required if
    a. There is residual first metatarsophalangeal joint (MTPJ) incongruence after the completion of the chevron osteotomy.
    b. There is a congruent joint but the lateral sesamoid lies wrapped around the lateral aspect of the first metatarsal (ie, fibrosed to this position and did not relocate during the chevron osteotomy displacement). This situation is found usually in elderly patients and in case of severe deformity.

The soft-tissue release involves a dorsal incision over the lateral recess of the first MTPJ using the Beaver blade. The blade is then inserted in a plantar direction into the plantar plate between the lateral sesamoid and the P1 base (lateral head of flexor hallucis brevis/sesame-phalangeal ligament). The Beaver blade is then rotated laterally at the same time as gently drawing the hallux into varus so that this ligament is

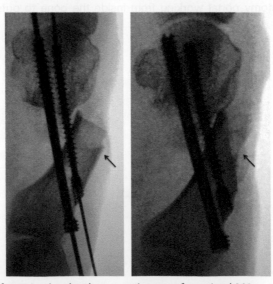

Fig. 7. Removal of proximal redundant prominence of proximal M1.

cut. The lateral collateral ligaments are not cut during this procedure. There is little excursion of the Beaver blade during this maneuver. The flexor hallucis longus is not at risk as long as the blade is positioned as described (**Fig. 8**).

Akin osteotomy

12. The decision as to whether to proceed to an Akin osteotomy depends on the degree of displacement of the preceding chevron osteotomy as well as the degree of hallux valgus interphalangeus. With greater chevron displacements (with or without internal rotation of the head fragment), an Akin osteotomy is less likely to be required.

    The Akin osteotomy is performed using a 12-mm Shannon burr via a medial mid-axial portal, which is positioned from a surface marking perspective midway between the hallux interphalangeal and MTPJs; this results in an osteotomy position at the junction of the diaphysis and the proximal metaphysis of the hallux. Once this position has been identified, the burr is inserted through the medial cortex of the phalanx but not through the lateral cortex. The burr is then rotated in both a dorsal and plantar direction to complete the Akin osteotomy (**Fig. 9**). The lateral wall is left intact apart from the dorsolateral and plantar lateral corners of the phalanx, which should be cut; otherwise, the osteotomy does not close. Because the burr is 2 mm in diameter, approximately 2 to 3 mm of bone is removed by the burr, essentially creating a slot that can then be closed. If further correction is required (very unusual), then the osteotomy is closed and the cut repeated in the same manner.

13. To fix the Akin osteotomy, a 3-mm screw is used via a medial portal proximal to the base of the P1. The guidewire is first inserted, and then when a satisfactory position has been achieved, the usual cannulated drilling and screw insertion can take place. The guidewire is then removed, and all the portals thoroughly irrigated with saline to remove any debris.

14. No sutures are required to the skin portals, but Redfern uses Steri-Strips on these. Saline- or chlorhexidine-soaked gauze is then applied (surgeon preference). These wet gauze dressings dry fairly hard and provide the patient with a comfortable and supportive dressing during the first 2 weeks before routine outpatient review at that stage. The dressings are completed with application of wool and crepe bandages.

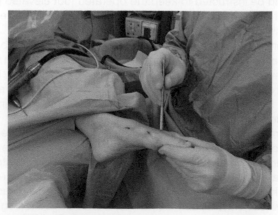

Fig. 8. Percutaneous distal soft-tissue release.

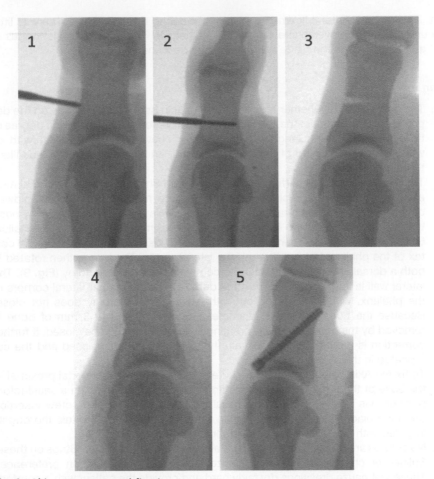

Fig. 9. Akin osteotomy and fixation.

Postoperative Care

The patient should be instructed to keep the operated foot elevated (above hip level) for 45 minutes of every hour for the first 2 weeks but to mobilize regularly for short periods during this time.

The patient is instructed on calf exercises for venous thromboembolism (VTE) prophylaxis, and a below-knee venous compression stocking is worn on the contralateral leg for the first 2 weeks postoperatively. VTE chemoprophylaxis may be prescribed in cases of bilateral correction if the patient has other risk factors such as obesity (apply local guidelines). No increase in complications has been observed in cases in which bilateral procedures have been undertaken.

The patient can be allowed to full weight bear immediately postoperatively in a stiff-soled surgical shoe (crutches provided for stability). The shoe must be worn at all times when weight bearing for the first 6 weeks after surgery. The first postoperative review (wound review) takes place at 2 weeks postsurgery, and all bandages and dressings are removed at that stage to inspect the portals. No further bandaging or splinting is required from 2 weeks onward, and the patient is encouraged to begin mobilizing the first MTPJ. Physiotherapy is usually recommended from 6 weeks onward to restore normal gait but is rarely required to restore first MTPJ motion, as stiffness is uncommon after this procedure as long as the patient begins mobilizing the joint at 2 weeks postsurgery as instructed. The patient is reviewed again at 6 weeks postsurgery with standing AP and lateral radiographs to ensure position has been maintained. The patient can then be allowed to return to his or her own footwear but can expect some limitation of choice of footwear for several months because of swelling. Patients can usually expect swelling to completely resolve within 4 to 6 months from surgery (**Fig. 10**). Running or racket sports are not allowed until 3 months postsurgery for big displacements (50%–100% displacement), but nonimpact sports are allowed from 6 weeks for all (eg, cycling, swimming, cross-trainer).

Further outpatient review takes place at 4 to 6 months postsurgery and at 1 year.

Complications

It is mandatory that any surgeon intending to take up this or any other percutaneous/minimally invasive technique seek appropriate cadaveric training from a surgeon experienced in these techniques before embarking on this surgery.

The list of potential complications is the same as for open hallux valgus surgery, which are well described. The main potential pitfalls for this technique are the following:

1. Poor positioning and execution of the chevron osteotomy. The surgeon must compensate for the slot that the burr cuts in the bone, both in terms of avoiding inadvertent elevation and shortening of the first metatarsal. The compensation for this is in the plane of the osteotomy (directed distally and plantarward as described in the technique section of this article).
2. Regular image intensifier views in both AP and lateral planes are essential during the procedure to ensure correct plane of osteotomy displacement and fixation.
3. Stable and reliable fixation can be relied on only if the screw fixation technique described earlier is followed. It is important that the proximal screw achieves 3-point fixation (ie, the proximal screw passes through the lateral cortex of the metatarsal proximal to the osteotomy and then continues on into the metatarsal head). Otherwise, there is insufficient angular control of the osteotomy during the postoperative period. and displacement achieved intraoperatively may not be maintained and might result in malunion.

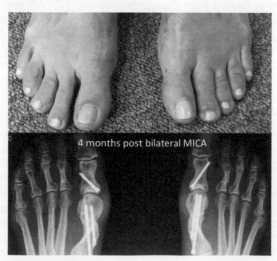

4 months post bilateral MICA

Fig. 10. MICA 4 months postsurgery.

Results and Evolution of Technique

Redfern, Vernois, Perera, and Lam have presented early results with the MICA technique at the British, German, Australian, and American Foot and Ankle Societes.[12–15]

But there are still little peer-reviewed published data. These data will emerge as experience grows, and early results with this technique seem encouraging with at least equivalent deformity correction, decreased postoperative stiffness, and reduced pain levels observed in comparison with open chevron and Scarf techniques.

Redfern and Walker presented their learning curve and early results with this technique in 2010. Seventy consecutive patients (83 osteotomies) were included in the study, and satisfactory improvements in intermetatarsal angles, hallux valgus angles, and Kitaoka scores were observed at 3 to 12 months follow-up. The investigators observed that 94% were either satisfied or very satisfied with the results of the surgery. Transfer metatarsalgia was observed in 4 patients, superficial infection in 2 patients, and no cases of deep infection, osteonecrosis, or nonunion. However, they observed a high rate of loss of fixation position during the postoperative period (7%) in this series, and 2 patients required further corrective surgery. This condition prompted Redfern and Vernois to recommend a change in the fixation technique to that which is described in this article, which has avoided this problem.

Redfern presented a larger series using the revised fixation method in 2014 at the DAF (Deutsche Assoziation für Fuß und Sprunggelenk e. V) Congress. He presented 125 feet (87 patients) with mean follow-up of 11.3 months (6–22 months). He did not observe any increased incidence of complications among the 38 patients who underwent bilateral surgery. He did not observe any cases of postoperative infection. Postoperative range of first MTPJ motion mirrored preoperative range. There were 3 malunions and 3 delayed unions but no nonunions or osteonecrosis, and overall, 96% of patients were either satisfied or very satisfied with the result. However, in 7% of feet, the distal screw became loose in the postoperative period such that it became prominent and had to be removed. This problem has been abolished with the new flanged-head screw design that was subsequently introduced.

As with open techniques, there is a scarcity of comparative data. In 2013 Perera[16] presented his early learning curve experience of MICA in a comparative study of MICA versus open chevron osteotomies (AOFAS 2013). He observed significantly better MOxFQ (Manchester Oxford Foot Questionnaire) and AOFAS scores in the MICA group than in the open chevron group. He also observed a lower infection rate as well as less post-operative pain and less stiffness in the MICA group. Similarly encouraging results were reported by Lam in a randomized comparative study between MICA and Scarf techniques presented at the American and British society meetings in 2014.

DISTAL MINIMALLY INVASIVE METATARSAL OSTEOTOMIES

The Weil osteotomy has been the main surgical workhorse for treating abnormalities of metatarsal cascade/imbalance of load distribution across the forefoot. However, this operation, although broadly adopted by foot and ankle surgeons, has a high incidence of postoperative stiffness and floating toe.[17,18] It is also difficult (if not near impossible) to correctly calculate the ideal/desired length and sagittal profile of the lesser metatarsals with this technique. Although the work of Maestro and colleagues[19] has been widely adopted as a method for calculating appropriate metatarsal length and hence position of fixation for Weil osteotomies, it does not take into account the sagittal plane of the metatarsal (metatarsal inclination) or other factors relevant in terms of the ideal position, such as the overall architecture of the foot, ankle motion, gastrocsoleus tension and the functional needs of the individual patient (eg, footwear). Khurna and colleagues[20] demonstrated the importance of metatarsal sagittal inclination in explaining failures after Weil osteotomy.

The idea of fixing all osteotomies rigidly with internal fixation has been indoctrinated into all modern foot and ankle surgeons, and although this makes sense if one is sure that the position of fixation is correct, it does not make sense in the case of lesser metatarsal osteotomies for the reasons outlined earlier.

Distal minimally invasive metatarsal osteotomies (DMMOs) have gained popularity in Europe as an alternative surgical technique to Weil osteotomy, partly because of the problems with stiffness and floating toe observed with the Weil osteotomy and partly because of the potential advantages of the dynamic correction offered by this technique. These osteotomies are performed via tiny portals at the distal diaphyseal-metaphyseal junction of the lesser metatarsals using a Shannon burr (2 × 12 mm) at an angle of 45° to the plane of the metatarsal.

Indications/Contraindications

The indications are the same as for the Weil osteotomy in the treatment of metatarsalgia. Surgeons vary in their threshold to use Weil osteotomies in such situations. The authors previously used the Weil osteotomy sparingly and although they now perform the DMMO instead, the indications are similarly narrow. An example would be metatarsalgia associated with hallux valgus in which adequate plantarisation of the first metatarsal head can usually obviate the need for surgery to the lesser metatarsals.

Contraindications also mirror those for Weil osteotomy and include active infection and insufficient vascular perfusion. However, DMMO's can often be considered in situations where the soft tissues of the forefoot are poor due to the percutaneous portal incisions rather than larger open incisions (as with the Weil), which may risk wound complications.

It is important to appreciate that when employing this technique there is a significant risk of a transfer lesions unless DMMO's are undertaken of the second, third and fourth metatarsals. A DMMO of the fifth should be added if there is a relatively small length difference between fourth and fifth metatarsals otherwise the patient might complain that the fifth toe does not sit comfortably against the fourth. Isolated DMMO's of a single metatarsal can be safely undertaken in certain circumstances but only when well experienced with this technique.

Surgical Technique

1. Equipment (see MICA)
   Burr: 2 × 12-mm Shannon burr
   Tourniquet: Not required and may encourage thermal injury to the soft tissues as the cooling effect of hemorrhage at the portals is lost
2. Anesthesia (either general or regional is administered) and intravenous antibiotics as per local guidelines
3. Positioning: The patient is positioned supine with the feet either on (if combining with open surgery) or overhanging the end of the operating table. The mini C-arm is positioned to the right of the patient regardless of which foot is being operated on (left side for left-handed surgeon)

Distal minimally invasive metatarsal osteotomy

1. When undertaking percutaneous surgery, the surgeon must learn to use the NDH as an additional navigation tool. In the case of DMMOs, the NDH is used to define

and protect the lesser MTPJ (**Fig. 11**). The thumb of the NDH is placed on the dorsal surface of the MTPJ (of the lesser metatarsal to be osteotomized) such that it covers the MTPJ and with it the dorsal articular surface of the metatarsal. The index finger of the NDH is placed on the plantar surface of the MTPJ so the surgeon essentially has the MTPJ between the thumb and index finger (see **Fig. 11**). With the dominant hand, a transverse stab incision is made with the Beaver blade to the right-hand side of, and adjacent to, the MTPJ (left side if left handed) (see **Fig. 11**). The stab incision is skin deep only. No deepening of the incision or periosteal elevation is required and might risk damaging the blood supply to the metatarsal head.

2. The 12-mm Shannon burr is then inserted through this portal directed extracapsularly toward the right-hand side of the metatarsal neck (left if left handed). The burr is then firmly rasped along the neck of the metatarsal proximally and distally (excursion of no more than a centimeter) so as to ensure the burr is on the bone and to locate the distal stop point on the neck where the burr abuts capsule of the MTPJ on the distal flare of the metatarsal neck (**Fig. 12**). This is the starting point of the osteotomy. Having located this, the surgeon must then orientate the burr such that it sits 45° dorsal to the metatarsal axis. The surgeon can confirm correct positioning of the burr on an image intensifier, but when more experienced, this will not be necessary.

3. The burr is then run (low speed) and engaged in the right-hand side of the metatarsal neck (maintaining sagittal 45° angle to the metatarsal axis). Once the burr has engaged the bone, the surgeon supinates the wrist in a smooth action until the burr lies flat on the foot at 90° to the metatarsal axis in the AP plane (**Fig. 13**). When performing a DMMO of the second metatarsal, the surgeon also needs to perform a sawing motion during this maneuver, as the burr is frequently not quite long enough to cut the metatarsal in 1 sweep otherwise. The osteotomy always finishes on the dorsal metatarsal surface (just proximal to the NDH thumb and hence remaining extra-articular).

4. If the surgeon is right-handed, then it is easiest to begin with the fourth metatarsal DMMO in the left foot and to then do the third and then second. This allows the fourth to fall out of the way before doing the third and so on. In the right foot, it is easiest for a right-handed surgeon to begin with the second metatarsal, then third, and then fourth.

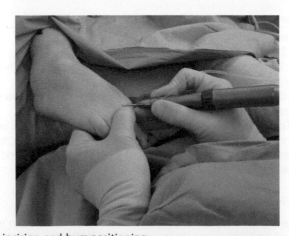

Fig. 11. DMMO incision and burr positioning.

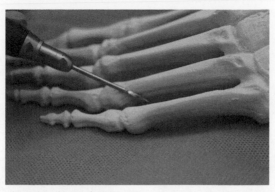

Fig. 12. Position and angle of burr for DMMO.

5. Once complete, the osteotomy should be mobile in the sagittal plane but should also telescope proximal-distal. If both these planes of motion are not present, then the osteotomy is not complete and the surgeon must replace the burr in the osteotomy to find where the intact bone remains, which must then be cut.
6. Finally, the lesser toes should be strapped with dressings to control/prevent the tendency for lateralization. Wet strips of gauze are preferred and used to strap each to the medial column of the foot (**Fig. 14**).

Postoperative Care

Patients should be instructed to keep the operated foot elevated (above hip level) for 45 minutes of every hour for the first 2 weeks but to mobilize regularly for short periods during this time. They should be told to expect the preoperative plantar pain (metatarsalgia) to be immediately abolished, but pain may be felt on the dorsum of the foot instead during the first 2 weeks after surgery. They may also experience some clicking in the forefoot due to movement of the osteotomies. As this is a dynamic correction,

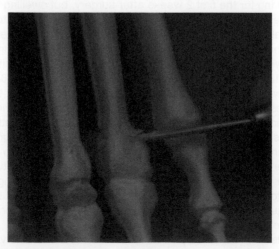

Fig. 13. Completion position of burr for DMMO.

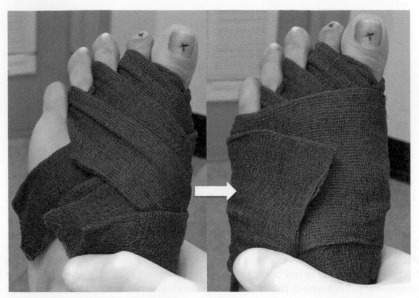

Fig. 14. Dressings technique in DMMO.

some weight bearing on the operated foot is important to set the functional position of the metatarsal heads, and the patient must understand this.

The patient is instructed on calf exercises for VTE prophylaxis, and a below-knee venous compression stocking is worn on the contralateral leg for the first 2 weeks postoperatively. VTE chemoprophylaxis may be prescribed in cases of bilateral correction where the patient has other risk factors such as obesity (apply local guidelines). No increase in complications has been observed in cases in which bilateral procedures have been undertaken.

The patient can be allowed to full weight bear immediately postoperatively in a stiff-soled surgical shoe (crutches provided for stability). The shoe must be worn at all times when weight bearing for the first 2 weeks after surgery, but swelling can dictate that the patient requires this shoe for several weeks beyond this. First postoperative review (wound review) takes place at 2 weeks postsurgery, and all bandages and dressings are removed at that stage to inspect the portals. No further bandaging or splinting is required from 2 weeks onward, and the patient is encouraged to begin mobilizing the lesser MTPJs. Physiotherapy is usually recommended from 4 to 6 weeks onward (depending on swelling) to restore normal gait but is rarely required to restore MTPJ motion, as stiffness is uncommon after this procedure as long as the patient begins mobilizing the joints at 2 weeks postsurgery as instructed. The patient is reviewed again at 6 weeks postsurgery with standing AP and lateral radiographs to ensure position has been maintained. The patient can then be allowed to return to his or her own footwear but can expect some limitation of choice of footwear for several months because of swelling. Patients can usually expect swelling to completely resolve within 4 to 6 months from surgery. Patients can be allowed to increase their activity level as guided by their symptoms but no sport before 3 months postsurgery to allow the osteotomies to consolidate.

Further outpatient review takes place at 4 to 6 months and at 1 year postsurgery **(Fig. 15)**.

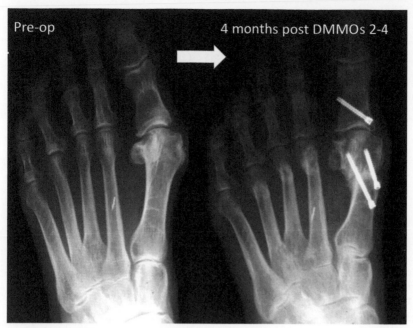

Fig. 15. DMMOs preoperation and 4 months postoperation.

Complications

It is mandatory that any surgeon intending to take up this or any other percutaneous/minimally invasive technique seek appropriate cadaveric training from a surgeon experienced in these techniques before embarking on this surgery.

The list of potential complications is the same as for any osteotomy, including infection (<0.5%), delayed/nonunion, malunion, and soft-tissue complications.

The risk of symptomatic nonunion is low (in the region of 1:500 to 1:1000), but delayed union is in the region of 5%. It is more common to see this in the second metatarsal osteotomy than more laterally. Delayed union is something the patient should be warned of preoperatively (bone union taking between 6 and 12 months to occur). Most of the delayed union cases unite within 6 to 12 months without any further treatment, and symptoms are usually mild (typically some aching discomfort in the dorsum of the foot in the region of the osteotomy and mild swelling in the same region). If troublesome, then placing the patient in a short removable surgical boot may encourage more rapid union, as these are usually hypertrophic delayed unions. If there is an atrophic appearance at 6 months postsurgery, then consider biological causes of delayed union as with any open osteotomy.

Malunion with this technique is, by open rigidly fixed surgical expectation, fairly high. It is fairly common for some lateral displacement of DMMOs of the second and third metatarsals, the fourth normally remains neutral, and the fifth (if performed) always displaces medially. This is due to the forces exerted by the flexors and extensors of the toes (**Fig. 16**). In addition, the surgeon should be cautious of using DMMOs in the presence of simultaneous hallux valgus correction, as the lateralization of the first metatarsal head tends to increase the tendency for the lesser metatarsal heads to displace laterally and can also result in some early recurrence of the hallux valgus unless strapping is used postoperatively. However, by strapping the lesser toes

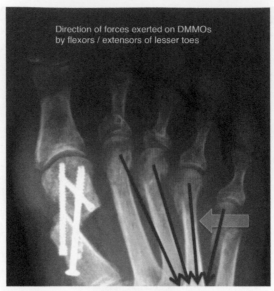

Fig. 16. Direction of soft-tissue forces acting on DMMOs.

medially to the medial column, this tendency for the lesser metatarsal heads to laterally displace (and externally rotate) is minimized, and any such displacement is rarely a clinical problem.

The main potential pitfalls for this technique are the following:

1. Soft-tissue (portal) complications. The skin over the dorsum of the foot is fragile. It is imperative that the surgeon adhere to the advised technique with low burr speed (<300 rpm) and high torque (50–80 Ncm) to avoid thermal injury to the skin surrounding the portal. Careful technique to ensure that the portal remains the center of rotation of the burr during the osteotomy also prevents mechanical injury to the portal.
2. Poor positioning of skin portal, which then results in the osteotomy being made in the wrong position. If the osteotomy is more proximal, then the lever arm on the osteotomy is greatly increased and the predominant mode of displacement is dorsal rotation at the osteotomy site, resulting in overelevation of the metatarsal heads. The intended position of the osteotomy should be checked on image intensifier before proceeding with the cut when inexperienced with this technique.
3. Poor plane of osteotomy. If the surgeon does not complete the DMMO with the burr perpendicular to the metatarsal axis, then an oblique osteotomy is created, which can encourage subsequent malunion. In experienced hands, adding some planned obliquity to the DMMO can be used to discourage undesired movement of the metatarsal head.

Results

Comparative literature is still lacking, but available studies suggest at least equivalent efficacy of DMMOs when compared with Weil osteotomies in the treatment of metatarsalgia.[21] The lack of postoperative stiffness is the main attraction with DMMOs, but the trade-off is almost certainly prolonged swelling in some patients and higher incidence of delayed union, although symptoms from this are usually low level. Symptomatic nonunion is rare (<1% in the experience of the authors).

TAILOR'S BUNION/BUNIONETTE

The treatment of bunionette deformity using these techniques is simple. A clinical classification of bunionette deformity is preferred over the traditional radiologic classification. The Redfern clinical classification divides these deformities into 2 groups:

Type I: The fifth toe is straight.
Type II: The fifth toe is in varus.

An additional element can be added (type Ia/IIa) to describe associated supination of the fifth toe. Treatment is based on the above-mentioned classification as follows.

Treatment of Redfern Type I Bunionette Deformity

A simple percutaneous shaving of the bunionette (prominent fifth metatarsal head) can be undertaken (**Fig. 17**). This procedure is performed via a dorsolateral stab incision portal 2.5 cm proximal to the lateral eminence of the fifth metatarsal head (**Fig. 18**). The straight elevator is then inserted and used to lift the capsule/periosteum from the lateral aspect of the fifth metatarsal head and create a safe working space. The 3.1-mm wedge burr is then inserted and used to shave the lateral aspect of the fifth metatarsal head under image intensifier guidance until sufficient reduction has been obtained. The bone debris is then washed out with saline using a syringe and cannula (the cannula is inserted up to the joint so that debris is flushed away from the joint in a retrograde direction). A rasp is used to remove any larger debris fragments from the surrounding soft tissue. No suture is required (Steri-Strip can be used), and a small dressing will suffice. The patient can full weight bear immediately and can usually return to normal footwear within the first few days postsurgery. Subsequent increase in patient activity can be dictated by comfort.

Treatment of Redfern Type II Bunionette Deformity

Appropriate treatment of these deformities requires a fifth metatarsal osteotomy (**Fig. 19**). A DMMO is almost always sufficient, but with severe widening of the 4/5

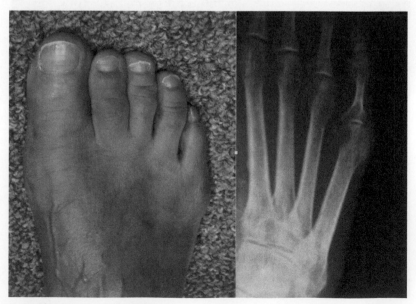

Fig. 17. Redfern type I bunionette.

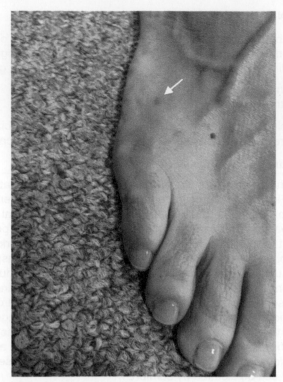

Fig. 18. Incision for bunionette shaving.

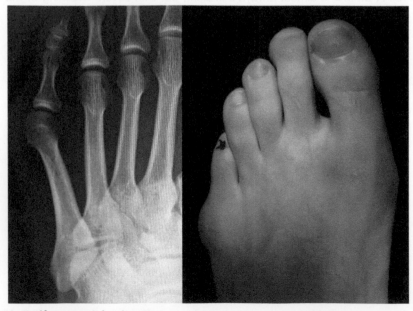

Fig. 19. Redfern type II bunionette.

intermetatarsal angle or severe banana deformity of the fifth metatarsal (severe type II and III by radiologic classification), the surgeon can use a more proximal closing wedge osteotomy if preferred. The DMMO is performed as described earlier in this article. Because the axis of the flexor and extensor tendons acts on the fifth toe, the fifth metatarsal head always displaces medially after a DMMO of the fifth metatarsal. No fixation is required, but postoperatively the foot can be taped simply (for 4 weeks) to maintain correction. With larger deformities and consequent larger head displacement after DMMO, it may be necessary to shave down the prominent lateral wall of the metatarsal diaphysis (**Fig. 20**), which can easily be performed with a 3.1-mm wedge burr via the same portal. The patient can full weight bear immediately and can usually return to normal footwear after the first postoperative week. Subsequent increase in patient activity can be dictated by comfort.

Treatment of Redfern Type Ia/IIa Bunionette Deformity

Treatment of these deformities begins with a derotation osteotomy of the fifth toe by performing a complete P1 osteotomy (at the proximal diaphyseal/metaphyseal junction) (see hammer toe section).

Treatment then proceeds as described earlier for the type I/II deformity. Postoperatively, the fifth toe is taped in the correct rotation for 4 weeks.

Complications

Complications are unusual. Delayed union is rare with DMMO of the fifth metatarsal, and Redfern has not encountered nonunion in this site with this technique. As described earlier, it is important to shave down the prominent lateral wall of the fifth metatarsal diaphysis (see **Fig. 20**) with larger displacements.

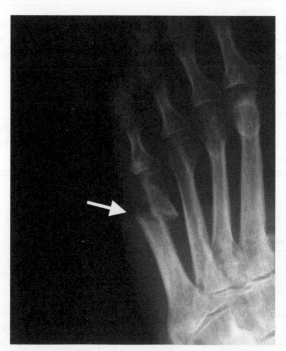

Fig. 20. Removal of prominent spike necessary with larger corrections.

If a more proximal medial closing wedge osteotomy is used for larger deformities (not necessary in the opinion of this author), then the surgeon should be aware of the risk of metatarsal elevation in the postoperative period due to the moment arm of forces acting at the site of the osteotomy.

LESSER TOE DEFORMITIES

Percutaneous surgical techniques are particularly suitable for the correction of lesser toe deformities and are particularly helpful in avoiding cutaneous or vascular complications (scar contracture, skin necrosis) in patients who might otherwise be at risk of such complications.

However, the main advantage is that these techniques afford the surgeon an almost limitless à la carte menu of surgical options, which can be tailored to a particular deformity. Percutaneous correction of these deformities allows targeted soft-tissue and bone procedures for different types of deformity and reducibility. Operative time savings should not be a the driving concern in embarking on these techniques because, although many flexible deformities can be corrected quickly, more complex and fixed deformities with or without subluxation/dislocation can take as long or longer than open surgical techniques.

Surgical Technique

1. Equipment (see MICA)
   Burr: 2 × 8-mm Shannon burr
   Tourniquet: Not required and may encourage thermal injury to the soft tissues, as the cooling effect of hemorrhage at the portals is lost. If undertaking these techniques with a tourniquet, then saline irrigation should be used
2. Anesthesia (either general or regional is administered) and intravenous antibiotics as per local guidelines
3. Positioning: The patient is positioned supine with the feet either on (if combining with open surgery) or overhanging the end of the operating table. The mini C-arm is positioned to the right of the patient regardless of which foot is being operated on (left side for left-handed surgeon)

The following surgical techniques are available:

1. Soft-tissue procedures
   a. Flexor tenotomies: Flexor digitorum brevis (FDB), flexor digitorum longus (FDL)
   b. Extensor tenotomies: Extensor digitorum longus (EDL), extensor digitorum brevis (EDB)
   c. Joint release: Metatarsophalangeal (MP), plantar proximal interphalangeal (PIP)
2. Bone procedures
   a. Extra-articular: Phalangeal osteotomy (P1, P2)
   b. Intra-articular: Condylectomy, condyloplasty, fusion (PIP, DIP)

Soft-Tissue Procedures

Flexor tendons
It is preferable to undertake only tenotomy of either the long or short flexor rather than both in any one toe.

Flexor digitorum brevis tenotomy for proximal interphalangeal flexion deformities This approach is proximal but adjacent to the interphalangeal (PIP) joint (**Fig. 21**). The incision is lateral or medial depending on the operated foot and according to the dominant hand of the surgeon. Plantar flexion of the toe during the

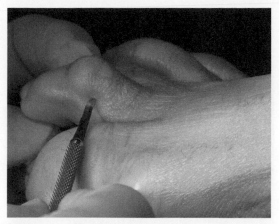

Fig. 21. Incision for FDB and plantar plate release.

procedure avoids injury to the plantar digital nerve with the Beaver blade during the procedure. The PIP joint plantar capsule is cut at the middle phalanx (P2) attachment and then the Beaver advanced more distally with a rotational movement for tenotomy of the two slips of FDB (**Figs. 22** and **23**). A periosteal elevator is then introduced to check that complete section of these slips has been achieved. The toe is then dorsiflexed at the PIP joint to confirm adequate release (**Fig. 24**).

An isolated FDB tenotomy may also be accomplished by plantar approach to the base of the P1 where the FDB lies superficially, but there is a higher risk of inadvertant section of the FDL also here. In addition, the plantar PIP release achieved by the PIP approach is helpful in correction of the stiff flexion deformities when present at this level.

Flexor digitorum longus tenotomy for distal interphalangeal flexion deformities The approach is a distal P2 plantar incision adjacent to the DIP joint but can also be performed with a lateral/medial incision, adjacent and proximal to the DIP joint. The toe is simultaneously dorsiflexed, which facilitates the tenotomy and allows the surgeon to feel when the tenotomy has been successfully completed.

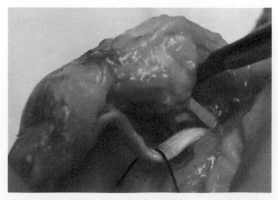

Fig. 22. Dissection showing position of blade in PIP joint and slips of FDB.

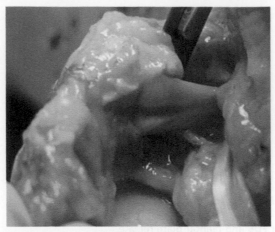

Fig. 23. Dissection showing blade releasing both slips of FDB.

Double flexor tenotomy (flexor digitorum longus + flexor digitorum brevis) This procedure was described by Mariano de Prado[10] and is performed via a proximal plantar P1 incision at the base of the toe (**Fig. 25**). Both FDL and FDB flexor tendons are sectioned, and completion of this maneuver is assessed by simultaneous dorsiflexion of the toe.

Extensor tendons

Extensor tenotomies for MP extension deformities are carried out in the area where the 2 tendons (EDL, EDB) are individualized (**Fig. 26**). If MP arthrolysis/capsulotomy is also required, then they can be tenotomized at the level of the MP joint but otherwise more proximally. Both EDL and EDB can be sectioned, or selective section can be undertaken if preferred. Simultaneous plantar flexion of the associated toe allows assessment of successful completion of the tenotomy, but this can often also be assessed visually in many feet (**Fig. 27**).

Joint release

Dorsal MP release (capsulotomy) is generally indicated only for MP dislocation and is the logical deep extension of the extensor tenotomies, but sometimes they are

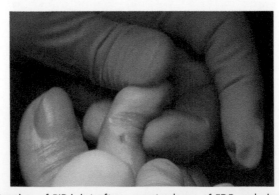

Fig. 24. Hyperextension of PIP joint after correct release of FDB and plantar plate.

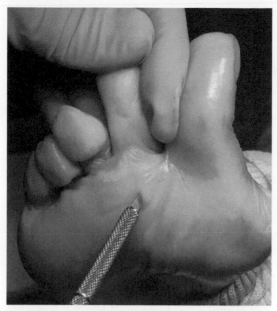

Fig. 25. Position of incision for double flexor tenotomy/P1 osteotomy.

laterally offset if there is associated varus or valgus deformity of the toe. Traction on the toe aligns and distracts the joint, facilitating the entrance of the Beaver blade when there is dislocation of the MP.

Performing indiscriminate dorsal MP capsulotomy in a normal or mildly subluxed MP can precipitate subsequent subluxation/dislocation of the MP, and the authors therefore recommend this procedure be reserved for cases of MP dislocation when such release is required as part of the surgical plan in achieving reduction of this joint.

Bone Procedures (Tailored to the Specific Deformity)

Extra-articular surgery
Proximal phalanx osteotomy This procedure is used to correct deformity at the MP joint and is performed via the same plantar approach as used for tenotomy of both flexor tendons (see **Fig. 25**). The osteotomy is optimally located at the proximal

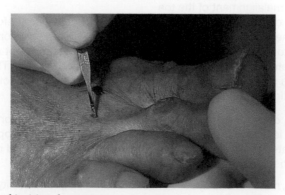

Fig. 26. Position of incision for extensor tenotomy.

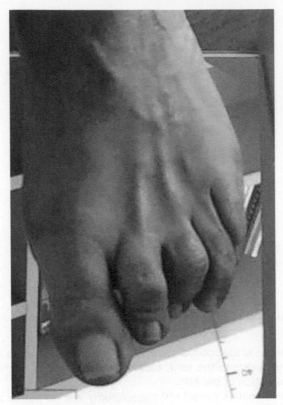

Fig. 27. Extensor tendons often easily visualized.

diaphyseal-metaphyseal junction region of the P1 or slightly proximal to this to optimize bone consolidation and to be as close as is safe to the level of deformity (MP joint). The osteotomy should not be made in the proximal/subchondral region of the metaphysis to avoid inadvertent intra-articular fracture or damage to the flexor tendons where they sit in the fibro-osseous groove on the plantar aspect of the P1 in this region. The osteotomy can be

1. Monocortical for plantar flexion correction of sagittal plane deformity or correction varus/valgus malalignment of the toe
2. Bicortical for deliberate shortening of the toe or more severe deformity (**Figs. 28** and **29**). An inexperienced surgeon may accidentally create a bicortical osteotomy when trying to create a monocortical osteotomy; this should not cause concern, but the osteotomy is less stable and may take longer to unite. The experienced percutaneous surgeon is also able to use oblique bicortical osteotomies to assist in the correction of the most severe triplanar deformities.

Middle phalanx osteotomy This procedure is used to correct deformity at the PIP level and/or DIP level and is achieved by a midaxial medial/lateral approach depending on the operated foot and the desired correction. It is performed middiaphysis to avoid damage to the PIP/DIP joints. The osteotomy can be

1. Monocortical, most commonly used to correct varus/valgus deformity of the distal toe (eg, clinodactyly) (**Figs. 30–33**) or to correct sagittal plane deformity in a stiff PIP joint

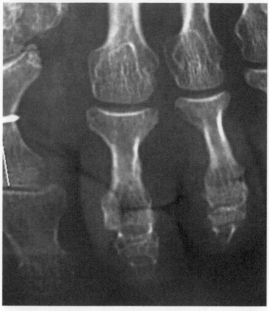

Fig. 28. Preoperative P1 osteotomy.

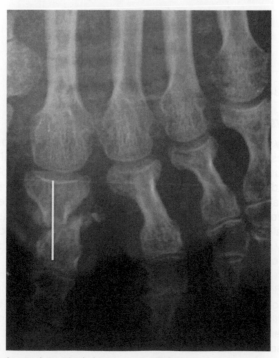

Fig. 29. Postoperative P1 bicortical shortening osteotomy.

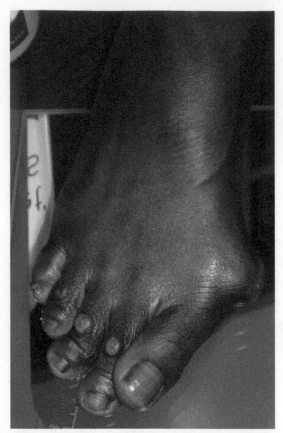

Fig. 30. Preoperative photograph of valgus deformity of the third toe.

2. Bicortical for deliberate shortening of the toe through the P2

Intra-articular surgery

1. Condylectomy is rarely required but can be performed via the P2 osteotomy portal. The purpose is to remove a prominent dorsal bump over the PIP joint when the surgeon has used a P1 and P2 osteotomy to correct, for example, a severe stiff hammer toe deformity. The condylectomy involves removing prominent bone from the dorsal aspect of the distal P1 and proximal P2. Bone debris is removed by pressure around the incision and then flushed away with saline (syringe and cannula). Residual bone debris may cause discomfort later in contact with the shoe. Condyloplasty can sometimes be easier performed using a distal dorsal approach level with the base of P2 (with the toe in plantar flexion).

2. PIP/DIP fusion can be performed via a midaxial medial/lateral incision directly over the joint. The 8-mm Shannon burr is used to denude both sides of the articular surface of cartilage and expose subchondral bone. Care should be taken to remove bone and cartilage debris, as this can create an unwanted inflammatory response in the postoperative period. The surfaces are then opposed, and the toe is stabilized with Kirschner (K) wires. Two 1-mm K-wires are preferred, as these can be cut and bent flush over the tip of the toe. Using 2 × 1-mm wires also controls

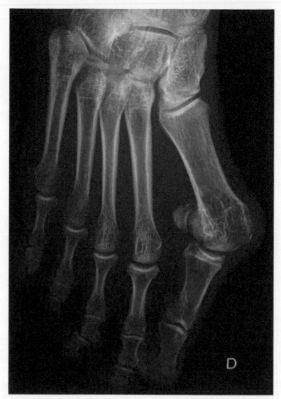

Fig. 31. Preoperative radiograph of valgus deformity of the third toe.

rotation, better preserving desired toe position, and reduces the incidence of infection during the postoperative period. It also allows the toe position to be altered after insertion of the wires (bending the wires) without making it difficult to remove them subsequently.

Indications: Which Percutaneous Surgery for Which Lesser Toe Deformities?

The decision as to which of the aforementioned techniques to use in any one particular lesser toe deformity is based on the morphology of the deformity and functional criteria and may also be influenced by the condition of the plantar plate and whether this is symptomatic.

Morphologic criteria
The surgeon needs to assess both sagittal (flexion/extension) and transverse (varus/valgus) plane deformity at each joint level.

In the case of PIP flexion deformity, the most frequent deformity at this level, the position of the DIP is variable and the MP may be neutral (hammer toe) or in dorsiflexion (claw toe).

Procedures used routinely for the correction of PIP flexion deformity are (**Figs. 34 and 35**):

- PIP plantar release and FDB tenotomy (if PIP is stiff)
- Plantar flexion P1 osteotomy. This procedure corrects deformity at the MP level, but if the extensor tendons are intact and the PIP joint is flexible, then as the

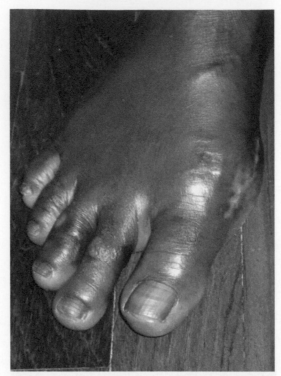

Fig. 32. Postoperative photograph of correction of valgus deformity of the third toe with P2 osteotomy.

osteotomy is closed, the extensor tendons act on the PIP and DIP joints to straighten them. Hence, routine extensor tenotomy in such circumstances is not recommended.

Less frequently required procedures for correction of PIP flexion deformity are

- Extensor tenotomy if the MP joint remains in extension despite use of the abovementioned routine procedures
- P2 osteotomy if the PIP joint correction is insufficient with the use of the abovementioned procedures (**Figs. 36** and **37**)

Functional criteria
The toe may be flexible, semirigid, or rigid. If the deformity is flexible, then generally, tenotomies can be avoided and bony surgery (osteotomy) will suffice. Rigid deformities often require a stepwise approach with soft-tissue surgery to create a more flexible situation before undertaking bony surgery in the form of phalangeal osteotomies. Intra-articular surgery is sometimes required depending on the circumstances.

Distal interphalangeal deformity

1. DIP flexion deformity: FDL tenotomy with or without P2 osteotomy (**Figs. 38** and **39**)
2. DIP deviation (varus/valgus) deformity: P2 monocortical osteotomy with closing wedge in the direction of desired correction. The osteotomy corrects the deviation without any need for DIP release (see **Figs. 30–33**)

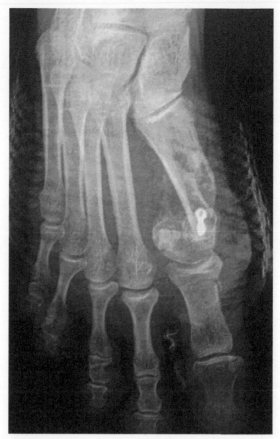

Fig. 33. Postoperative radiograph of correction of valgus deformity of the third toe with P2 osteotomy.

CONDITION OF THE PLANTAR PLATE

Piclet recommends the use of ultrasonography (dynamic examination)/MRI to assess the plantar plate if rupture is suspected. If confirmed, then she prefers to add a distal metatarsal osteotomy to the correction. She uses a DMMO if there is no radiographic subluxation of the MP joint but otherwise prefers to undertake a mini-open osteotomy with fixation.

Redfern does not routinely image the plantar plate as it is the clinical findings that guide his surgical algorithm.

Treatment of other particular scenarios
- Flexible distal deformities may benefit from isolated FDL tenotomy.
- Neurologic deformities are often sufficiently treated by tenotomy of both the flexors (FDL and FDB), for example, flexion dystonia deformities in Parkinson disease.
- Isolated extensor tenotomy may be sufficient in cases of MP extension without any PIP flexion deformity.
- Lateral deviation of the toes without flexion deformity is treated with an osteotomy of P1, often in combination with percutaneous distal metatarsal osteotomy (DMMO) (**Figs. 40–42**).

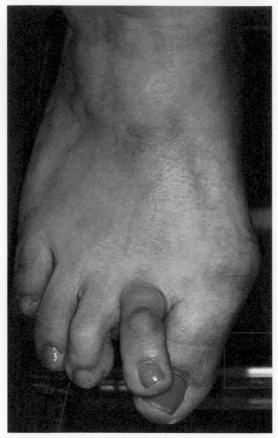

Fig. 34. Preoperative photograph of patient with varus deformity and PIP joint flexion deformity of the second toe.

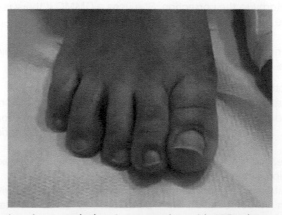

Fig. 35. Postoperative photograph showing correction with FDB release and P1 osteotomy.

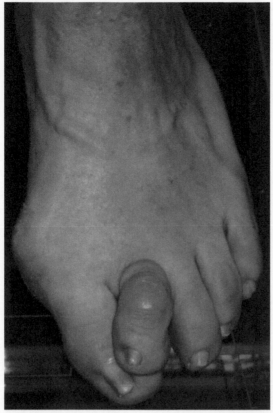

Fig. 36. Preoperative photograph of patient with varus deformity and PIP joint flexion deformity of the second toe.

- Isolated P1 osteotomy is often sufficient in flexible deformity of the third and fourth toes (**Figs. 43** and **44**).
- P2 isolated osteotomy is performed for clinodactyly (see **Figs. 30–33**).
- Iatrogenic or posttraumatic deformities with overlapping toes may require several phalangeal osteotomies (**Fig. 45**).

POSTOPERATIVE MANAGEMENT

The surgeon wishing to take up these techniques needs to learn how to control the toe position both in the immediate postoperative period (wet dressings applied in theater) and in the 6 weeks following surgery. There are various techniques of taping/strapping the toes once the dressings are removed at the first postoperative review, but essentially the toes must be controlled in the desired position until union has occurred (if using phalangeal osteotomies in the surgical correction).

The patient is allowed to full weight bear immediately after surgery but should keep the operated foot strictly elevated for the first 7 to 10 days. Initial postoperative review usually takes place at 1 week, with subsequent frequency of review depending on the procedures undertaken and the ability of the patient to manage the strapping/taping correctly. The surgeon should ensure that the taping/strapping is effective during the 6-week period following surgery to optimize the final result.

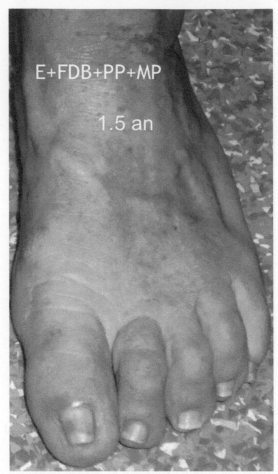

Fig. 37. Postoperative photograph showing correction with FDB release, P1 osteotomy, and P2 osteotomy.

Complications

Infection is rare after percutaneous lesser toe surgery. The risk of neurovascular injury is also low if the techniques are carried out carefully with respect to the anatomy and very low burr speeds. Some toe numbness can occur in the initial postoperative period but usually represents neuropraxia with return of sensation 4 to 6 weeks later. Incomplete correction, new deformity, or recurrence of deformity can occur if the surgeon does not ensure good technique of toe control with taping/strapping in the postoperative period (see earlier discussion).

Results

In 2009, Barbara Piclet presented her results with percutaneous lesser toe correction at the Second Congress of Minimally Invasive Surgery in Murcia. She presented the results of 112 feet that underwent second toe deformity correction involving FDB tenotomy, PIP release, and P1 osteotomy, with postoperative review at 6 and 36 months. She reported 97% patient satisfaction with 78% assessed as good

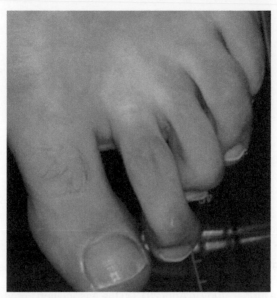

Fig. 38. Preoperative photograph of patient with mallet deformity of the second toe.

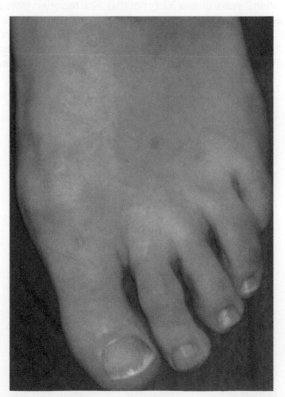

Fig. 39. Postoperative photograph showing correction of mallet deformity with FDL tenotomy and P2 osteotomy.

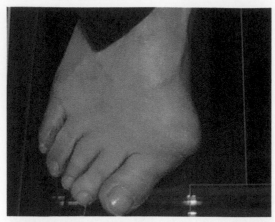

Fig. 40. Preoperative photograph of lateral/valgus deviation of the lesser toes.

correction and 19% with moderate but painless residual deformities. She observed recurrence in 3% of patients.

She presented a further study in April 2013 in the Association Française de Chirurgie du Pied with a prospective series of 57 feet that underwent percutaneous surgical correction of the second toe without any metatarsal surgery with a postoperative follow-up of more than 2 years (mean 30.7 months). She reported 90% patient satisfaction with the correction in all respects. About 98% of patients were happy with the cosmetic result, 98% were happy with improvement in footwear comfort, 75% reported no footwear restriction, and 77% patients were pain free. PIP flexibility was retained in 88% of cases, standing toe ground touch in 86%, and toe grasp present in 86%.

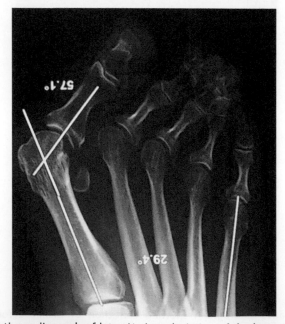

Fig. 41. Preoperative radiograph of lateral/valgus deviation of the lesser toes.

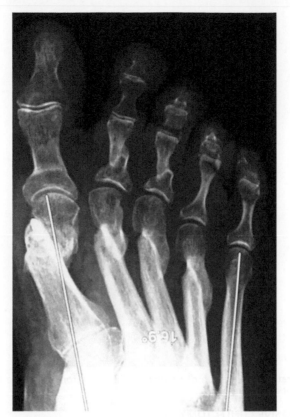

Fig. 42. Postoperative radiograph of correction of lateral/valgus deviation of the lesser toes using P1 osteotomy and DMMO.

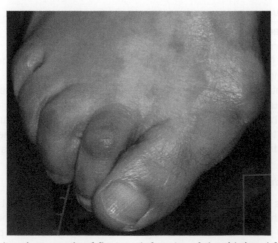

Fig. 43. Preoperative photograph of flexion deformity of the third and fourth toes.

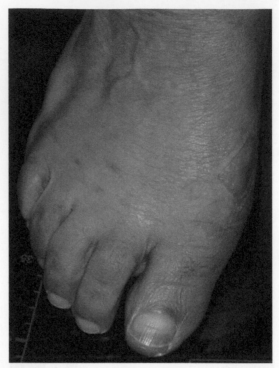

Fig. 44. Postoperative photograph of correction flexion deformity of the third and fourth toes with isolated P1 osteotomy.

MINIMALLY INVASIVE CHEILECTOMY

The results of open cheilectomy for hallux rigidus have been well documented in the literature.[22] The use of percutaneous techniques to undertake cheilectomy has dramatically reduced the morbidity of this procedure while still delivering comparable success in terms of outcome. Indications for this procedure are the same as for the open procedure.

Surgical Technique

1. Equipment (see MICA)
   Burr: 3.1-mm wedge burr
   Tourniquet: Not required and may encourage thermal injury to the soft tissues, as the cooling effect of hemorrhage at the portals is lost
2. Anesthesia (either general or regional is administered) and intravenous antibiotics as per local guidelines
3. Positioning: The patient is positioned supine with the feet overhanging the end of the operating table. The mini C-arm is positioned to the right of the patient regardless of which foot is being operated on (left side for left-handed surgeon)

Cheilectomy of the first metatarsophalangeal joint

1. The incision is made over the dorsomedial aspect of the first metatarsal (**Fig. 46**). This incision should be approximately 2.5 cm proximal to the MP joint so as to avoid damaging the portal during the burring of the osteophytes. If the portal is too low, then this creates difficulty in removing the osteophytes with the burr. Care should

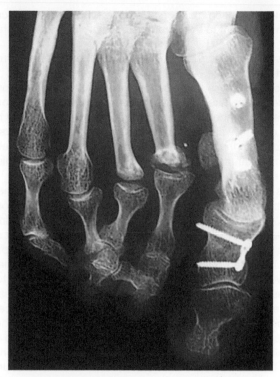

Fig. 45. Iatrogenic or posttraumatic deformities with overlapping toes may require several phalangeal osteotomies.

be taken to avoid damaging the dorsomedial cutaneous nerve during creation of the portal (and subsequently during the procedure) as it is close (portal should be just plantar to the nerve). The incision should be approximately 8 mm long to allow effective wash out of debris later in the procedure.

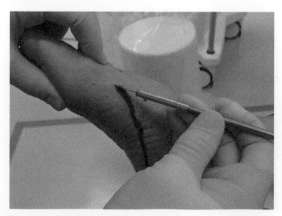

Fig. 46. Position of incision for cheilectomy.

2. Once the incision has been made, a straight elevator is used to create a working space up to and adjacent to the dorsal osteophyte (but not over the dorsal aspect of this).

3. The 3.1-mm wedge burr is then introduced via the portal and run at low speed (<300 rpm but high torque, eg, 80 Ncm) as it is engaged into the osteophyte (**Fig. 47**). The osteophyte is removed from inside out. The surgeon should not try and engage the osteophyte from the dorsal aspect, as this will possibly endanger the extensor hallucis tendons. Instead, the osteophyte is engaged by the burr at its base and then gradually pulverized working from the base in a dorsal direction and then more distally into the osteophyte and repeating until completely removed. The surgeon must not plantar flex the hallux during this process as this may place the hallux extensor tendons at risk of injury.

4. As progress is made in removal of the osteophyte, so it becomes necessary to remove debris; this is achieved by expressing the pulverized bone paste out of the portal (**Fig. 48**) and then flushing out further debris using a syringe and cannula (cannula is inserted up to the joint so that flushing is retrograde). Larger fragments of bone debris can be removed from the soft tissues using a rasp.

5. The resection is carried out with image intensifier guidance. When experienced, very little x-ray is required, as the surgeon can feel the osteophyte with the NDH, and this guides progress with the burr. However, it is always essential to obtain a lateral image intensifier view (**Fig. 49**) at the end of the procedure to ensure that no bone debris has been left in the region of the resection. Any hint of opacity dorsal to the resection on these views should alert the surgeon to the likelihood of substantial residual debris remaining and the need for further washout and rasping to clear this. If this debris is not fully cleared, then it can incite an unwanted inflammatory response in the postoperative period.

6. The amount of bone resected depends on the surgeon's preference, but the dorsal 30% is usual and 90° of dorsiflexion at the MP should be possible at the end of the procedure.

Removal of P1 osteophytes

7. If P1 osteophytes are present and are a possible source of impingement, then these can be removed by simply advancing the burr into the dorsal metaphysis of the P1 and continuing the resection as for the metatarsal osteophyte.

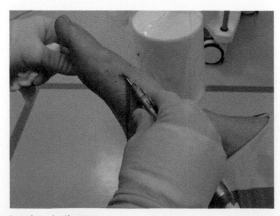

Fig. 47. Burr insertion for cheilectomy.

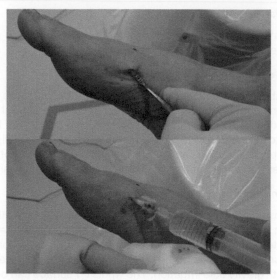

Fig. 48. Washout and rasping of cheilectomy debris.

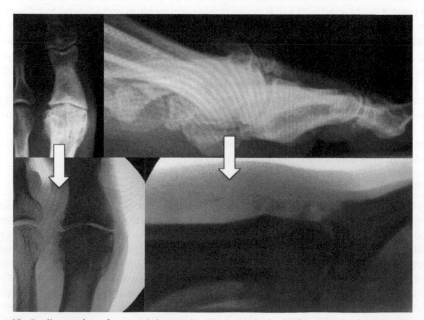

Fig. 49. Radiographs of pre–minimum incision surgery cheilectomy and post–minimum incision surgery cheilectomy.

Removal of medial metatarsal osteophytes

8. If medial metatarsal osteophytes are present, then these can be removed via the same dorsomedial portal.

Removal of lateral metatarsal osteophytes

9. If lateral metatarsal osteophytes are present, then these can be removed via an additional lateral portal at the same level as the dorsomedial portal but to the lateral side of the extensor hallucis tendon. Once the skin portal has been made, the straight elevator is inserted straight onto bone and then slid distally until it encounters the osteophyte. The burr then follows the same path, and both lateral M1 and P1 osteophytes can easily be removed (and washed out in a similar manner).

Optional additional arthroscopy

10. It is helpful to augment the cheilectomy with arthroscopy of the MP joint to inspect the resection (especially if inexperienced with percutaneous cheilectomy), assist with adequate washout, and deal with synovitis and loose chondral fragments. This procedure is undertaken using the 4-mm arthroscope via the initial dorsomedial portal with gravity fluid irrigation. The whole P1 surface can be inspected with this portal, and a shaver can be introduced via a dorsolateral portal at the level of the joint to remove synovitis/chondral flaps as required. To view the entire M1 surface, an additional medial midaxial portal is made at the level of the joint through which the arthroscope can be inserted (adjacent to the joint but not into the joint space).
11. The portals are closed with Steri-Strips, and simple dry dressing is applied with wool and crepe bandaging.

Postoperative Management

The patient is provided with a stiff-soled postoperative shoe and allowed to full weight bear immediately but instructed to keep the foot elevated for most of the first 72 hours. Patients can remove the bandages at home at 24 hours postsurgery (leaving the dressing in place, however) and can return to their own footwear at 4 days postsurgery. They are instructed to begin simple active range of motion exercises of the hallux MP joint from day one. First postoperative outpatient review (wound review) takes place at 1 week postoperatively, and the portals have usually healed by that stage. The patient then begins physiotherapy, which is directed at restoration of normal gait and range of motion in the hallux MP joint. The patient is instructed to refrain from sport or long periods of weight bearing activity for the first 4 weeks but then allowed to return to full activity as their symptoms dictate.

Results

As yet there is little published data relating to results from minimally invasive cheilectomy. Redfern undertook a retrospective study (David Redfern, FRCS[Tr&Orth], unpublished data, 2014) looking at 44 consecutive feet (39 patients, male/female = 9:30) undergoing percutaneous cheilectomy for hallux rigidus. The mean preoperative AOFAS score was 63 (35–80), and hallux dorsiflexion (HDF) was 39° (0°–80°). Mean follow-up was 9 (6–13) months. Postoperatively, the mean AOFAS score was 77 (65–100) and HDF 56° (30°–90°). Outcome was reported as very satisfactory in 26 of 44 feet, with mean reported subjective percentage improvement in symptoms (SPI) of 90% (75%–100%). In 9 of 44, satisfactory outcome and SPI of 72% (60%–80%) were reported. Outcome was disappointing in 11 feet with SPI of

33% (0%–50%). One patient underwent subsequent fusion surgery. About 86% of patients returned to ordinary footwear and normal daily activity/employment by 1 week postsurgery. There were no superficial or deep infections, and only 1 patient reported numbness in the hallux laterally.

Complications

Infection is a rare complication of this technique. Dorsomedial cutaneous nerve injury is a small risk (<3%). The authors have not encountered extensor tendon injury using this technique.

REFERENCES

1. Hymes L. Introduction: brief history of the use of minimum incision surgery (MIS). In: Fielding MD, editor. Forefoot minimum incision in podiatric medicine: a handbook on primary corrective procedures on the human foot using minimum incisions with minimum trauma. New York: Futura Pub Co; 1977. p. 1–2.
2. Wilson D. Treatment of hallux valgus and bunions. Br J Hosp Med 1980;24:548–9.
3. Bosch P, Wanke S, Legenstein R. Hallux valgus correction by the method of Bosch: a new technique with a seven-to-ten year follow-up. Foot Ankle Clin 2000;5:485–98.
4. Isham S. The Reverdin-Isham procedure for the correction of hallux abductovalgus. A distal metatarsal osteotomy procedure. Clin Podiatr Med Surg 1991;8:81–94.
5. Reverdin J. De la deviation en dehors du gros orl (hallux valgus) et son traitement chirurgical. Tran Int Med Congress 1981;2:408–12.
6. Magnan B, Bortolazzi R, Samaila E, et al. Percutaneous distal metatarsal osteotomy for correction of hallux valgus. Surgical technique. J Bone Joint Surg Am 2005;88(Suppl 1 Pt 1):135–48.
7. Giannini S, Vannini F, Faldini C, et al. The minimally invasive hallux valgus correction "S.E.R.I." Interact Surg 2007;2-1:17–24.
8. Bauer T, de Lavigne C, Biau D, et al. Percutaneous hallux valgus surgery: a prospective multicenter study of 189 cases. Orthop Clin North Am 2009;40(4): 505–14, ix.
9. Siclari A, Decantis V. Arthroscopic lateral release and percutaneous distal osteotomy for hallux valgus: a preliminary report. Foot Ankle Int 2009;30(7):675–9.
10. De Prado M, Ripolli PL, Golano P. Minimally invasive foot surgery: surgical techniques, indications, anatomical basis. Bilbao (Spain): About Your Health; 2009. ISBN 8461316096, 9788461316090.
11. Kelikian H. Hallux valgus. In: Mann RA, Coughlin MJ, editors. Allied deformities of the forefoot and metatarsalgia. Philadelphia: WB Saunders; 1965. p. 213–25.
12. Vernois J. The treatment of the hallux valgus with a percutaneous chevron osteotomy. J Bone Joint Surg Br 2011;93(Suppl IV):482.
13. Redfern D, Gill I, Harris M. Early experience with a minimally invasive modified chevron and akin osteotomy for correction of hallux valgus. J Bone Joint Surg Br 2011;93(Suppl IV):482.
14. Walker R, Redfern D. Experience with a minimally invasive distal lesser metatarsal osteotomy for the treatment of metatarsalgia. Orthopaedic Proceedings 2012;94B:39.
15. Vernois J, Redfern DJ. Percutaneous chevron; the union of classic stable fixed approach and percutaneous technique. Fuss & Sprunggelenk 2013;11(2):70–5.
16. Redfern D, Perera AM. Minimally invasive osteotomies. Foot Ankle Clin 2014; 19(2):181–9.

17. Hofstaetter SG, Hofstaetter JG, Petroutsas A, et al. J Bone Joint Surg Br 2005; 87(11):1507–11.
18. Beech I, Rees S, Tagoe M. A retrospective review of the Weil metatarsal osteotomy for lesser metatarsal deformities: an intermediate follow-up analysis. J Foot Ankle Surg 2005;44(5):358–64.
19. Maestro M, Besse JL, Ragusa M, et al. Forefoot morphotype study and planning method for forefoot osteotomy. Foot Ankle Clin 2003;8(4):695–710.
20. Khurna A, Kadamabande S, James S, et al. Weil osteotomy: assessment of medium term results and predictive factors in recurrent metatarsalgia. Foot Ankle Surg 2011;17(3):150–7.
21. Henry J, Besse JL, Fessy MH, et al. Distal osteotomy of the lateral metatarsals: a series of 72 cases comparing the Weil osteotomy and the DMMO percutaneous osteotomy. Orthop Traumatol Surg Res 2011;97(Suppl 6):S57–65.
22. Hattrup SJ, Johnson KA. Subjective results of hallux rigidus following treatment with cheilectomy. Clin Orthop Relat Res 1988;(226):182–91.

Fifth Metatarsal Osteotomies

Lowell Weil Jr, DPM[a],*, Devon Consul, BSN, RN[b]

KEYWORDS

- Bunionette • Osteotomy • Scarfette • Tailor's bunion

KEY POINTS

- A tailor's bunion or bunionette deformity is a combination of an osseous and soft tissue bursitis located on the lateral aspect of the fifth metatarsal head.
- A variety of surgical osteotomy procedures has been described for the bunionette deformity.
- Metatarsal osteotomies of the 5th metatarsal narrow the forefoot, maintain the length of the metatarsal, and preserve function of the metatarsophalangeal joint.

INTRODUCTION

A tailor's bunion or bunionette deformity is a combination of an osseous and soft tissue bursitis located on the lateral aspect of the fifth metatarsal head, and was first described by Davies[1] as a condition caused by splaying of the fifth metatarsal. The condition is often present with hallux valgus deformity, both of which are noted with a flexible splayfoot (**Fig. 1**).

Chronic shoe pressure over the lateral part of the fifth metatarsal head leads to hypertrophy of the overlying soft tissue; bursal thickening; and, less often, localized hyperkeratosis. In the presence of hallux valgus deformity, the width of the forefoot is increased, thereby causing increased pressure on the lateral side of the fifth metatarsal head. The cause of the deformity of the fifth metatarsal head can be a localized, enlarged bony prominence but most often the cause is a rotational movement of the fifth ray at its articulation with the cuboid. The fifth ray excessively pronates, leading to a progressive deformity that is accompanied by the fifth toe seeking an adductovarus position.[2–4] The condition can also occur as a result of a structural deformity with both plantar flexion and abduction of the fifth ray, producing a plantar keratosis as well as a bunionette deformity. The plantar keratosis condition is most frequently seen in a cavus foot type.[5]

As in hallux valgus deformity, several retrospective studies indicate that the condition is between 3 and 10 times more common in women than in men and has

Disclosure: The authors have nothing to disclose.
[a] Weil Foot & Ankle Institute, 1455 Golf Road, Des Plaines, IL 60016, USA; [b] Dr. William M. Scholl College of Podiatric Medicine, 3333 Green Bay Road, North Chicago, IL 60064, USA
* Corresponding author.
E-mail address: lwj@weil4feet.com

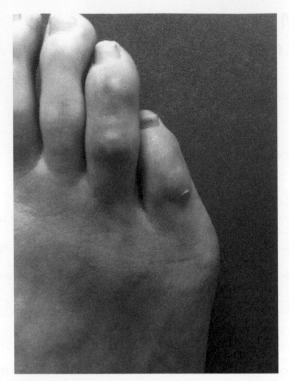

Fig. 1. Classic bunionette deformity.

a peak incidence during the fourth and fifth decades of life.[2,6] Conservative treatments may resolve some of the associated bursitis or fifth metatarsal-phalangeal joint, but are not likely to create any long-term benefits.[2]

SURGICAL PLANNING

In 1990, Fallat and Bucholz[7] described a classification system for surgical management of symptomatic tailor's bunion. Type 1 is an enlargement of the lateral aspect of the fifth metatarsal head; type 2, a lateral bowing of the distal aspect of the pronated fifth metatarsal; type 3, an increased fourth-fifth intermetatarsal (IM) angle; and type 4, a combination of 2 or more deformities. Coughlin[8] postulated that these criteria should enable the surgeon to better recognize the type of bunionette deformity and assist in the choice of an appropriate surgical technique.

A key radiographic measurement associated with a bunionette deformity is the IM angle between the fourth and fifth metatarsals, which normally averages 4.5°.[2,7] This finding usually relates to the fifth metatarsal prominence distance (protrusion of the lateral metatarsal head surface from the shaft, measured by a line drawn along the lateral cortex of the fifth metatarsal shaft and another line drawn along the lateral cortex of the fifth metatarsal head; normal <4 mm)[9]; 4-5 metatarsal head distance (distance between the lateral cortex of the fourth metatarsal head and the medial cortex of the fifth metatarsal head; normal <3 mm)[10]; and the fifth metatarsal plantar-declination angle (horizontal bisection of the fifth metatarsal in relation to the weight-bearing surface; normal 108°).[2] The normal length of the fifth metatarsal is considered to be 12 mm shorter than the fourth metatarsal, producing a gentle oblique taper from the central metatarsals in a lateral direction.[2] These findings and observations allow surgeons to make the determination and selection of the appropriate surgical osteotomy procedure.[2] One additional observation that should be considered is the position of the bony prominence, keratosis, or bursitis on the fifth metatarsal head, namely dorsolateral, lateral, or plantar-lateral. This important finding may influence the decision of which surgical procedure is best indicated.[11] For example, a plantar keratosis may benefit from a procedure that elevates the metatarsal head along with angular correction; a fifth metatarsal cheilectomy rather than an osteotomy may be appropriate in a case with primarily dorsolateral prominence.

SURGICAL DECISION MAKING FOR BUNIONETTE DEFORMITY

The guidelines for bunionette surgery at the Weil Foot & Ankle Institute are presented here.

In some cases, the prominent dorsal or dorsolateral aspect of the fifth metatarsal head is the symptomatic area and the IM angle is normal. In these cases, without large bunionette deformity, a simple dorsal-lateral cheilectomy is sufficient to alleviate symptoms and an osteotomy is not needed. However, most cases with a bunionette show a 4-5 IM angle in excess of 6°. In these cases, an osteotomy is indicated. Our algorithm calls for either a Weil osteotomy (WO), as suggested by Barouk,[12] or a short scarfette osteotomy with an IM angle between 5 and 8°. The WO is commonly recommended because of its inherent stability in the sagittal plane, technical ease, and rapid healing. In the case of an intractable plantar keratosis, a scarfette osteotomy is the procedure of choice because of its ability to correct the deformity and elevate the head, diminish plantar pressure, and remain stable during healing.

As the IM angle and bowing of the fifth metatarsal increase, the scarfette is carried more proximal, allowing for greater surface area for bony healing and stability (**Figs. 2** and **3**). It is never longer than 50% of the length of the fifth metatarsal and we are careful to stay away from the proximal metadiaphyseal region to avoid any potential for nonunion in that area. In cases of a plantar flexed fifth metatarsal head, as seen in a cavus foot, the long scarfette (**Fig. 4**) allows for dorsal as well as medial translation to render a more favorable position.

When we encounter a failed case of bunionette correction, we prefer a metatarsal arthroplasty and remove a few millimeters to a full centimeter from the distal articular surface and perform a plantar condylectomy. This method shortens the toe but it is a final correction of the deformity that renders a rapidly healing procedure for a challenging situation.

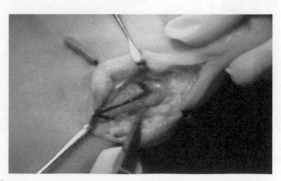

Fig. 2. Short scarfette.

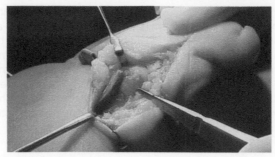

Fig. 3. Short scarfette displaced 5 mm.

SURGICAL OSTEOTOMY PROCEDURES

Medial oblique sliding osteotomy (with fixation)
Medial, oblique slide osteotomy; minimally incision procedure (no fixation)[3,13]
SERI (simple, effective, rapid, inexpensive[14]; with fixation)
Chevron (distal osteotomy with or without fixation)[2–4]
Closing, lateral wedge osteotomy at metatarsal neck or proximal diaphysis[2,3,15]
WO[12]
Scarfette[3,11,12]

MEDIAL OBLIQUE SLIDING OSTEOTOMY

In 1971, Smith and Weil[16] published a technique article on a medial oblique sliding osteotomy of the fifth metatarsal head using an osteotome to create the osteotomy. This osteotomy was performed through a 1-cm incision overlying the metaphyseal area of the metatarsal area (**Fig. 5**). The 12-mm osteotome was positioned so that an angle was formed of 70° from distal-lateral to proximal-medial and undercut by 15°. The purpose of this angle was to have the bone slide medially with little chance of lateral subluxation. The undercut of the metatarsal head helped to avoid dorsal migration of the head following surgery. A dressing was applied, bandaging the fifth toe in an abducted position to ensure medialization of the metatarsal head. Patients were advised to maintain guarded weight bearing for 1 week. The results were good with respect to ultimate cosmetic appearance but chronic swelling and 3 to 4 months of healing were necessary for complete resolution.

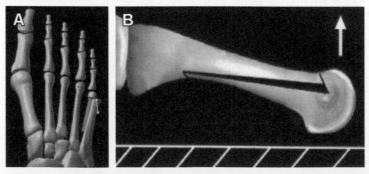

Fig. 4. (*A*, *B*) Long scarfette osteotomy; Long scarfette allows for dorsal as well as medial translation to render a more favorable position. (*A*) allows for observation of the medial translation component (*arrow*) and (*B*) allows for observation on the dorsal translation component (*arrow*). Weil 1984 (short), Barouk 1995 (long).

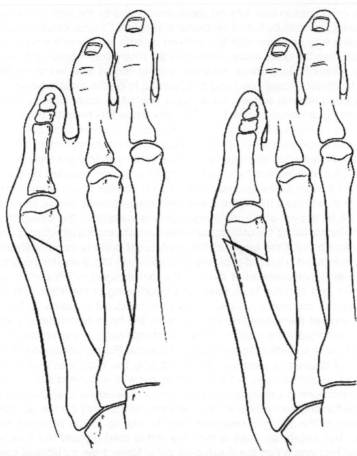

Fig. 5. Oblique sliding osteotomy of the fifth metatarsal. (*From* Smith SD, Weil LS. Fifth metatarsal osteotomy for tailor's bunion deformity: minor surgery of the foot. Mt Kiscoe (NY): Futura; 1971.)

MINIMAL INCISION SURGERY

Bunionette correction via an osteotomy through a minimal incision may be performed using several methods. Probber and White[13] popularized the procedure. Under a local anesthetic, a puncture incision was made at the lateral metaphysis of the flare of the fifth metatarsal head.[13] A dental cutting burr was used to create a blind osteotomy at a 90° angle to the metatarsal shaft. Some minimal incision surgeons used fluoroscopy to verify intraoperative position. The cut allowed mobilization of the fifth metatarsal head in a medial direction to correct the deformity. The bone debris (paste) caused by the high-torque/low-speed burr was extirpated through the dermal opening and the wound irrigated and closed with a single 6-mm (quarter-inch) Steri-Strip (3M Nexcare Products, St Paul, Minnesota). No fixation was used and a compression dressing was applied, bandaging the fifth toe in an abducted position to ensure medialization of the metatarsal head. Patients were permitted to ambulate immediately and return to work as needed. Retrospective, uncontrolled results of the procedure were published with short-term follow-ups. However, personal observations of our senior partner (Lowell Scott Weil, Sr, 1991) were remarkably good with respect to clinical outcome but with a high complication rate. Wound problems caused by the heat of the rotary burr usually healed uneventfully but some became infected. Chronic swelling lasting up to 3 to 5 months was common with this unfixed osteotomy. Nonunion was infrequent, perhaps because the bone paste created by the rotary burr facilitated healing of the osteotomy. Uncontrolled, dorsal elevation was observed that led to metatarsalgia under the fourth metatarsal head and this seemed to be the most adverse complication that needed revision surgery. Most cases yielded an acceptable cosmetic result with no scarring or dorsal contracture. The procedure has recently become popular with orthopedic surgeons in Spain, France, and Italy. However, because of the limited outcomes and studies available, and the tendency for dorsal malunion, it is difficult to routinely recommend this technique until more extensive data are reported.

An alternative mini-incision technique using fixation was reported by Giannini and colleagues.[14] A 1-cm lateral incision is made just proximal to the lateral eminence of the fifth metatarsal head through the skin and subcutaneous tissue, down to bone. Once the lateral aspect of the metatarsal neck is visualized, the osteotomy is performed. The inclination of the osteotomy in the lateral to medial direction is perpendicular to the fourth ray if the length of fifth metatarsal bone is to be maintained. The osteotomy is inclined in a distal-proximal direction up to 25°, if shortening of the metatarsal bone or decompression of the metatarsophalangeal (MTP) joint is desired in cases of mild joint arthritis. More rarely, if a lengthening of the fifth metatarsal bone is necessary, the osteotomy is inclined in a proximal-distal direction up to 15°.

After creation of the osteotomy with the saw, the head is mobilized with a small osteotome and medial translation of the metatarsal head is performed introducing the Kirschner wire superficial to the lateral eminence. Plantar translation of the metatarsal head, if desired, is produced by introducing the Kirschner wire in the upper aspect of the metatarsal head. A 1.8-mm Kirschner wire is inserted into the soft tissue adjacent to the bone in a proximal to distal direction along the longitudinal axis of the fifth toe. The Kirschner wire exits at the lateral area of the tip of the toe, adjacent to the lateral border of the nail; it is retracted with the drill up to the proximal end of the osteotomy. The metatarsal head is then translated medially and the Kirschner wire is advanced retrograde into the diaphyseal canal toward the metatarsal base. If the cut edge of the metatarsal is laterally prominent, a small wedge of bone is removed. The skin is sutured with a single 3-0 stitch. The Kirschner wire is bent and cut at the tip of the toe. Ambulation is allowed immediately using a postoperative shoe that allows weight bearing only on the hindfoot. After 1 month, the dressing, suture, and Kirschner wire are removed. Patients are allowed to return to normal comfortable shoe wear, and gentle exercises with cycling and swimming are advised (**Fig. 6**).

Giannini and colleagues[14] reported that 48 of 50 patients were satisfied with their results. The preoperative American Orthopaedic Foot and Ankle Society (AOFAS) forefoot score was 62.8 ± 15.1 points (range, 19–80 points) and postoperatively it was 94 ± 6.8 points (range, 75–100 points) ($P<.0005$). Thirty-eight feet (76%) were rated as excellent, 9 (18%) good, 2 (4%) fair, and 1 (2%) was considered poor. Pain was absent in 40 feet (80%), mild or occasional in 8 feet (16%), and moderate or daily in 2 feet (4%). Function in 42 feet (84%) had no limitations in daily and sport activities; 7 feet (14%) had minimal limitations; and 1 foot (2%) had a severe limitation. Forty-four patients (88%) were able to wear normal shoes.

All osteotomies had healed radiographically at an average of 3 months. All the osteotomies remodeled over time, even in cases with significant offset initially. Radiographic evaluation showed that the average fifth MTP angle was $16.8° \pm 5.1°$ preoperatively and $7.9° \pm 3.1°$ ($P<.0005$) postoperatively. The 4-5 IM angle was $12° \pm 1.7°$ preoperatively and $6.7° \pm 1.7°$ postoperatively ($P<.0005$). No severe complications, such as avascular

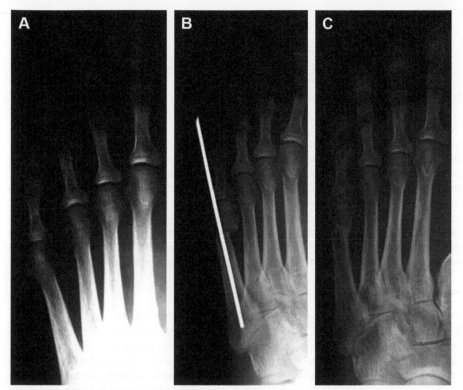

Fig. 6. (*A–C*) Giannini and colleagues' SERI procedure.

necrosis of the metatarsal head or nonunion of the osteotomy, occurred. In 6 feet (12%), the radiographic healing of the osteotomy occurred more than 4 months after surgery. However, no increased postoperative pain was noted in these patients, and the clinical result was not compromised at final follow-up. Furthermore, no correlation was found between the delayed radiographic union and the offset at the osteotomy; none of these cases displaced. One foot (2%) had a skin inflammatory reaction around the Kirschner wire. Two feet (4%) reported symptomatic plantar callosities under the fourth metatarsal heads. No dorsal subluxation of the fifth MTP was present. Further studies with larger numbers of patients, longer follow-up, determination of the risk of dorsal malunion or metatarsalgia, and stratification for severity of deformity are necessary before recommending this procedure on a widespread basis.

CHEVRON OSTEOTOMY

Following the success of a stable construct for the Austin (chevron) hallux bunionectomy, several investigators,[2] including Kitaoka and Holiday,[4] used a similar technique for the bunionette deformity. Through a dorsal or lateral incision, a lateral exostectomy was performed on the fifth metatarsal head removing a small amount of bone. A chevron osteotomy was then performed in the cancellous bone of the metatarsal head (**Figs. 7** and **8**). The head was mobilized and translated medially by about 3 to 6 mm (**Figs. 9** and **10**). Using manual compression, the fifth metatarsal head was firmly compressed from distal to proximal (**Fig. 11**). The lateral overhanging ledge that remained was carefully resected so as to not interrupt the osteotomy position. Later,

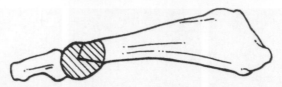

Fig. 7. Chevron osteotomy for bunionette correction.

some surgeons chose to use fixation with a Kirschner-wire to avoid malunion and delayed healing (**Figs. 12** and **13**). At present, surgeons routinely use absorbable pins or small-diameter screws for fixation (**Fig. 14**). Guarded weight bearing was recommended and most patients had a very favorable outcome. Healing usually took 2 to 3 months for resolution of swelling, and the cosmetic appearance was good. However, in larger deformities with a 4-5 IM angle greater than 8°–10°, the width of the fifth metatarsal head did not allow enough medial displacement to reduce the deformity adequately. As such, this may be a good option for smaller deformities or cases with outflaring of the distal metatarsal shaft that do not require such a large correction.

PROXIMAL CLOSING WEDGE OSTEOTOMY

In 1972, Gerbert and colleagues[15] presented preliminary results of a fifth metatarsal shaft osteotomy described as a long oblique wedge resection. A dorsal incision measuring 4 to 5 cm in length is placed directly overlying the fifth metatarsal neck and shaft from the fifth metatarsal to the junction between the proximal and middle one-third of the fifth metatarsal. The incision is deepened directly through the skin to the level of the capsule and periosteum overlying the fifth metatarsal neck and shaft. A long oblique osteotomy was outlined from distal-medial to proximal-lateral and terminating at the junction of the lateral shaft and base of the fifth metatarsal. The osteotomy was performed in such a manner as to maintain the proximal-lateral cortical-periosteal hinge. A small 2-mm to 3-mm medially based wedge of bone was then resected from the proximal and medial portion of the fifth metatarsal and

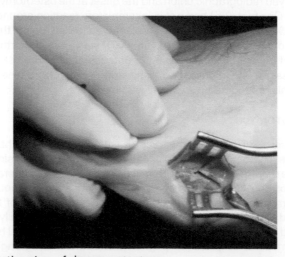

Fig. 8. Intraoperative view of chevron osteotomy.

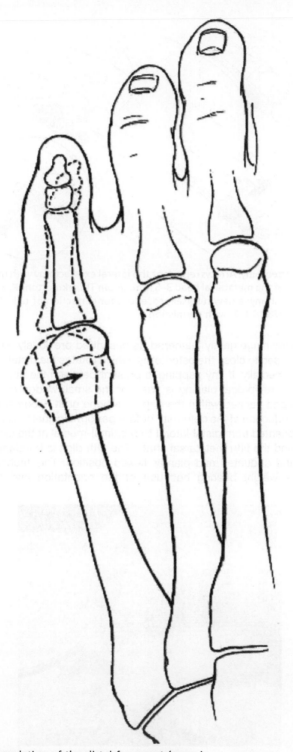

Fig. 9. Medial translation of the distal fragment (*arrow*).

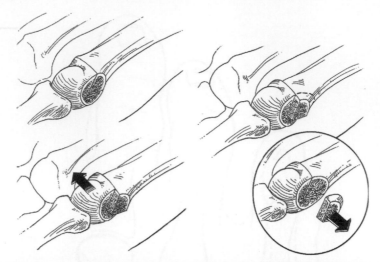

Fig. 10. Chevron osteotomy. Arrows represent the lateral exostectomy with mobilization and medial translation of the metatarsal head 3–6 mm. (*From* Throckmorton JK, Bradlee N. Transverse V sliding osteotomy: a new surgical procedure for correction of tailor's bunion deformity. J Foot Surg 1978;18:117; with permission.)

the proximal-lateral hinge gently feathered as described previously (**Fig. 15**). A small bone clamp was used to close the osteotomy, which rotates the distal fifth metatarsal, capital fragment medially. If any gapping is present between the distal and proximal capital fragments, reciprocal planing is used or the small wedge of bone resected then morselized and packed within the gap as a bone graft. Fluoroscopy is used to verify complete reduction of the deformity before performing final fixation with a small, oblique screw, oriented from distal-lateral to proximal-medial at the junction between the osteotomy and the fifth metatarsal shaft. The fifth digit is bandaged in a slightly overcorrected and abducted and plantar flexed position. This technique does not allow immediate weight bearing because of the orientation and fragility of the

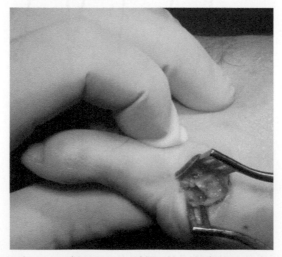

Fig. 11. Manual translation and impaction of head on shaft.

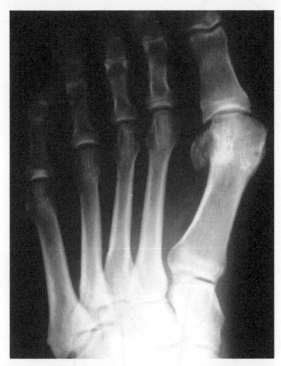

Fig. 12. Preoperative view of bunionette.

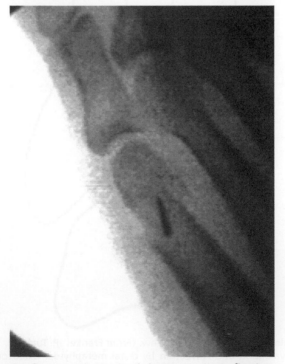

Fig. 13. Intraoperative fluoroscopic image of chevron with pin fixation.

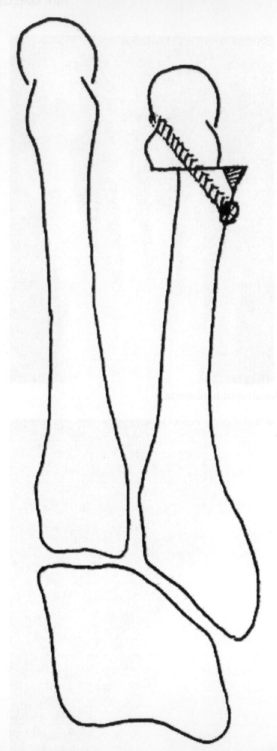

Fig. 14. Absorbable pin. Small-diameter screw. (*From* Frankel JP, Turf RM, King BA. Tailor's bunion: clinical evaluation and correction by distal metaphyseal osteotomy with cortical screw fixation. J Foot Surg 1989;28(3):237–43; with permission.)

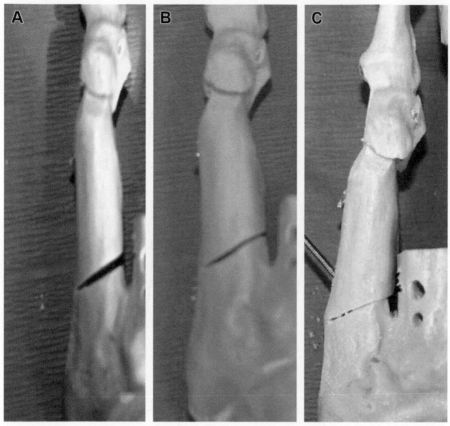

Fig. 15. (A–C) Closing medial wedge at neck and oblique shaft osteotomy for bunionette deformity.

osteotomy and, therefore, should be protected non–weight bearing in either a short-leg cast or removable immobilization boot. Serial radiographs are obtained to monitor osseous healing and, once verified, the patient is allowed to return to a roomy athletic or Oxford shoe with weight bearing to tolerance. This stage can occur from 6 to 8 weeks. Castle and colleagues,[17] in a retrospective review of 26 long oblique wedge resection osteotomies, found a mean IM 4-5 angle reduction of 1.58 (7.9–6.48) and a mean lateral deviation angle reduction of 3.98 (4.1–0.28). One osteotomy fractured following a traumatic incident in the early postoperative period but there were no reported incidences of delayed union, malunion, or transfer lesions. This osteotomy seems most useful for the correction of an abnormally large IM 4-5 angle.

Coughlin[8] describes a sliding oblique midshaft osteotomy to correct increased IM 4-5 angle and/or increased lateral bowing (**Figs. 16–18**).[2,8] Several cases of nonunion and delayed unions have been noted with this procedure, probably from inadequate weight bearing or patient noncompliance.

WEIL OSTEOTOMY

Barouk[12] recommends the WO for small to intermediate deformity because of the inherent stability and ease of performing this procedure (**Fig. 19**). However, like the chevron procedure, it has limitations in the narrow metatarsal head.

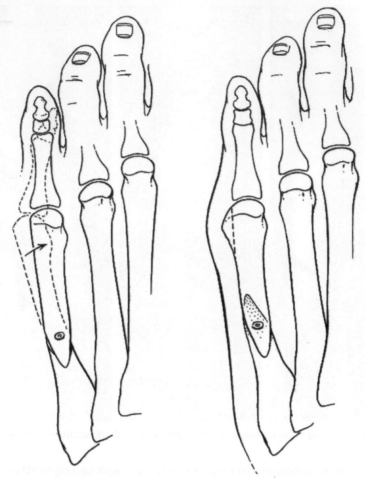

Fig. 16. Sliding oblique midshaft osteotomy. Arrow allows for visualization of the correction of the increased IM angle. (*From* Coughlin MJ. Correction of the bunionette with midshaft oblique osteotomy. Orthopedic Trans 1988;12:30–1; with permission.)

SCARFETTE OSTEOTOMY

Based on the favorable results of the scarf procedure for hallux valgus deformity, Weil[11] proposed a reverse scarf procedure for the bunionette deformity. Barouk[12] later popularized the procedure and gave it the name scarfette. The 3-cm, laterally based incision is carried directly through the capsule and periosteum, which are sharply reflected to expose the dorsal and plantar-lateral aspects of the fifth metatarsal head and neck. A minimal lateral exostectomy is performed with a power saw. The scarf-shaped cut about 2.5 cm long is outlined from dorsal-distal to plantar-proximal on the fifth metatarsal head and neck (**Fig. 20**). A 60° dorsal-distal osteotomy is performed 3 mm proximal to the articular cartilage of the fifth metatarsal head. Next, the central horizontal osteotomy directed from superior to inferior is performed with the saw held in slight dorsal angulation so as not to plantar displace the osteotomy fragment. Lastly, a proximal 60° plantar osteotomy is performed at the proximal plantar extent of the horizontal osteotomy (see **Fig. 2**). The neck of the fifth metatarsal shaft bows plantarly, so note that the proximal portion of the osteotomy

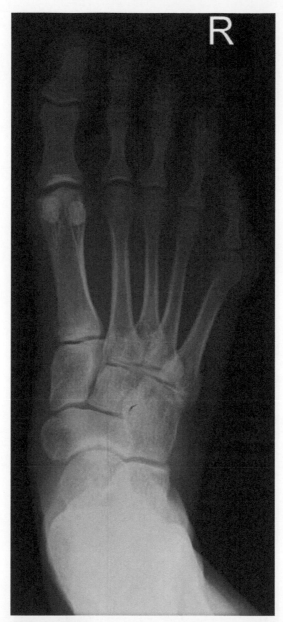

Fig. 17. Before Coughlin osteotomy.

does not end up at midshaft. It should be at the plantar one-third of the metatarsal shaft to avoid potential stress fracture. A small, thin osteotome is inserted in the osteotomy and gently rotated to verify completion of the osteotomy. With traction on the fifth digit, the fifth metatarsal head is gently manipulated in a medial direction to reduce the deformity. Once completed, a small clamp is placed on the lateral fifth metatarsal shaft and the osteotomy fragment. Fixation was initially performed with manual impaction and capsulorrhaphy but some cases developed displacement so fixation with a buried threaded 1.6-mm pin or 2.5-mm screw was used thereafter (**Figs. 21** and **22**). Once

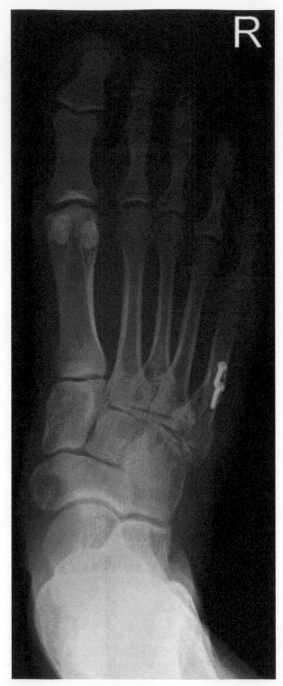

Fig. 18. After Coughlin oblique midshaft osteotomy.

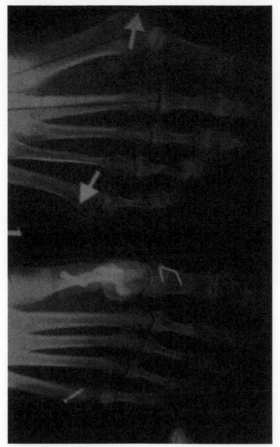

Fig. 19. Before and after WO of fifth metatarsal for bunionette. Arrows demonstrate the small to intermediate deformity prior to WO.

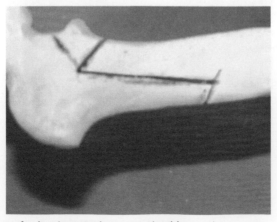

Fig. 20. Scarfette cut for bunionette (note proximal low cut).

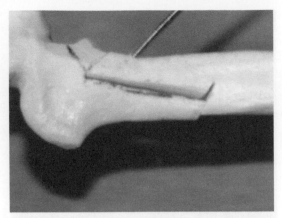

Fig. 21. Medial displacement; impact and fixate with threaded pin or screw.

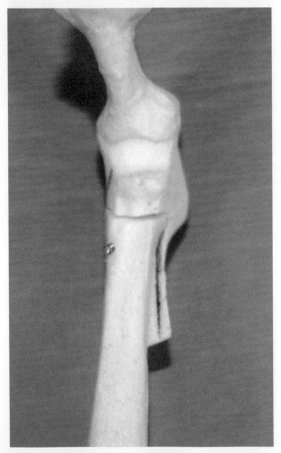

Fig. 22. Scarfette displacement with stable construct.

adequate correction is obtained, the osteotomy fragment is impacted on the metatarsal. The remaining lateral head, neck, and shaft is carefully removed and smoothed with power instrumentation. The periosteum and capsule are repaired with 3-0 absorbable suture. A running subcuticular stitch followed by Steri-Strips (3M Nexcare Products, St Paul, Minnesota) are used to repair the skin. The postoperative period was standard for each patient, and included a bulky dressing with the fifth toe bandaged in abduction and a surgical shoe with patients using guarded weight bearing immediately after surgery. At the first postoperative appointment 1 week later, all patients were transitioned into a running shoe and started physical therapy for strengthening and range-of-motion exercises.

Follow-up was performed in 50 patients at an average of 12 months.[18] The average age was 50.23 ± 14.31 years. There were 44 (88%) women and 6 (1.2%) men. The operative side included 27 (54%) right and 23 (46%) left feet. Preoperatively, the mean IM 4-5, lateral deviation angle (LDA) and fifth MTP joint angles were 10.34° ± 2.40°, 4.15° ± 4.08° and 15.56° ± 6.83° respectively. Nineteen (38%) patients had a type 2 deformity and 31 (62%) patients had a type 3 deformity. The 19 patients with a type 2 deformity had a mean LDA of 9.0° ± 3.46°. Postoperatively at 1 year, the mean IM 4-5, LDA, and fifth MTP joint angles were corrected to 1.80°± 2.21°, 0.24°± 0.46°, and 2.40° ± 7.94° respectively. Postoperative correction of the IM 4-5, LDA, and fifth MTP joint angles were statistically significant ($P<.001$). Complications included 1 undercorrection and 7 hardware removals.

Maher[19] reported on 63 patients who underwent operative repair of 77 tailor's bunion deformities with a scarfette technique between September 1999 and September 2006. Eighty-six percent were completely satisfied, 11.4% were satisfied with reservations, and 3% were dissatisfied. Ninety-one percent considered themselves better than before their surgery, whereas 8.6% thought that they were no better. Ninety-one percent of patients said they would undergo surgery under the same conditions again. Preoperatively, the mean 4-5 IM angle measured on weight-bearing radiographs was 9.9° (standard deviation [SD], 2.2), the mean postoperative IM angle was 5.7° (SD, 2.0). The mean preoperative AOFAS score was 44.1 points (SD, 14.5) and the mean postoperative score at 6-month review was 91.8 (SD, 20.2). The clinical improvement was maintained, with an AOFAS score at final review 36 months after surgery of 88.1 (SD, 11.6).

SUMMARY

A variety of surgical osteotomy procedures has been described for the bunionette deformity. Metatarsal osteotomies narrow the forefoot, maintain the length of the metatarsal, and preserve function of the MTP joint. Distal metatarsal osteotomies produce less correction and reduce postoperative disability; however, they pose a risk of inadequate correction because of the small width of the fifth metatarsal head and transfer lesions if shortened or dorsiflexed excessively. The sliding oblique metaphyseal osteotomy described by Smith and Weil[16] (without fixation) and later by Steinke and Boll[20] (with fixation) is easy to perform and provides good cancellous bone contact. Fixation is sometimes difficult and bone healing can take a few months because of the unstable construct of this osteotomy. Kitaoka and Holiday[4] describe a distal chevron osteotomy that provides lateral pressure relief and reduced plantar pressure. This osteotomy is currently the most common procedure used, but it may prove difficult to perform if the deformity is large and the bone is narrow. Diaphyseal osteotomies are indicated when greater correction is needed; however, they require more dissection and there is greater postoperative convalescence with non–weight bearing for several weeks. Proximal base osteotomies may be used to address significantly increased IM 4-5 angles or when a large degree of sagittal plane correction is required. Approaches that have been described include opening and closing base wedges and basal chevrons. Advantages to this approach are the ability to avoid epiphyseal plates in pediatric patients and maintenance of function of the MTP joint, whereas disadvantages include inherent instability of the location of the osteotomy, embarrassment of intraosseous and extraosseus blood supply of the metatarsal, and technical demand. Non–weight bearing is essential for several weeks. The scarfette procedure is a combination head-shaft procedure that is indicated to treat mild to moderate transverse and sagittal plane deformities.[11,18] The inherent stability of the osteotomy and ability for early weight bearing of the scarfette makes this our procedure of choice when selecting treatments for patients with a bunionette deformity.

ACKNOWLEDGMENTS

The authors thank T. Roukis, DPM, for his help with illustrations and photographs.

REFERENCES

1. Davies H. Metatarsus quintus valgus. Br Med J 1949;1:664–5 St Louis7 Mosby; 1993. p. 441–65.
2. American College of Foot and Ankle Surgeons. Tailor's bunion and associated fifth metatarsal conditions: preferred practice guidelines. Park Ridge (IL): American College of Foot and Ankle Surgeons; 1993.
3. Roukis TS. The Tailor's bunionette deformity: a field guide to surgical correction. Clin Podiatr Med Surg 2005;22:223–45.
4. Kitaoka HB, Holiday AD Jr. Lateral condylar resection for bunionette. Clin Orthop 1992;278:183–92.
5. Diebold PF. Basal osteotomy of the fifth metatarsal for bunionette. Foot Ankle 1991;12:74–9.
6. Hansson G. Sliding osteotomy for tailor's bunion: brief report. J Bone Joint Surg Br 1989;71(2):324.
7. Fallat LM, Bucholz J. Analysis of the tailor's bunion by radiographic and anatomic display. J Am Podiatry Assoc 1980;70(12):597–603.
8. Coughlin MJ. Treatment of bunionette deformity with longitudinal diaphyseal osteotomy with distal soft tissue repair. Foot Ankle 1991;11:195–203.
9. Karasick D. Preoperative assessment of symptomatic bunionette deformity: radiologic findings. AJR Am J Roentgenol 1995;164(1):147–9.
10. Nestor BJ, Kitaoka HB, Ilstrup DM, et al. Radiologic anatomy of the painful bunionette. Foot Ankle 1990;11:6–11.
11. Weil LS. The reverse scarf osteotomy for tailor bunion deformity. Seoul (Korea): SICOT; 1992.
12. Barouk LS. Some pathologies of the fifth ray: tailor's bunion. In: Barouk LS, editor. Forefoot reconstruction. Paris (France): Springer-Verlag; 2002. p. 276–83.
13. White DL. Minimal incision approach to osteotomies of the lesser metatarsals: for treatment of intractable keratosis, metatarsalgia, and tailor's bunion. Clin Podiatr Med Surg 1991;8(1):25–39.
14. Giannini S, Faldini C, Vannini F, et al. The minimally invasive osteotomy "S.E.R.I." (simple, effective, rapid, inexpensive) for correction of bunionette deformity. Foot Ankle Int 2008;29:282–6.

15. Gerbert J, Sgarlato TE, Subotnick SI. Preliminary study of a closing wedge osteotomy of the fifth metatarsal for correction of a tailor's bunion deformity. J Am Podiatry Assoc 1972;62(6):212–8.
16. Smith SD, Weil LS. Fifth metatarsal osteotomy for tailor's bunion deformity: minor surgery of the foot. Leander (TX): Futura Publishing; 1971.
17. Castle JE, Cohen AH, Docks G. Fifth metatarsal distal oblique wedge osteotomy utilizing cortical screw fixation. J Foot Surg 1992;31(5):478–85.
18. Glover J, Weil L Jr, Weil L Sr. Scarfette osteotomy for surgical treatment of bunionette deformity. Foot Ankle Spec 2009;2(2):73–8.
19. Maher AJ, Kilmartin TE. Scarf osteotomy for correction of tailor's bunion: mid- to long-term followup. Foot Ankle Int 2010;31(8):676–82.
20. Steinke MS, Boll KL. Hohmann-Thomasen metatarsal osteotomy for tailor's bunion (bunionette). J Bone Joint Surg Am 1989;71:423–6.

Metatarsus Primus Varus Correction

Matthew D. Sorensen, DPM, FACFAS[a],*, Brian Gradisek, DPM[a],
James M. Cottom, DPM[b]

KEYWORDS

- Metatarsus primus varus • Hallux valgus • Bunion
- Distal first-metatarsal osteotomy • Proximal metatarsal osteotomy • Lapidus
- SCARF bunionectomy correction • Apex of deformity

KEY POINTS

- The quest for definitive, irrefutable etiologic definition of the common hallux valgus foot deformity continues.
- To date, no all-encompassing theory or clinically proven entity has emerged to settle the debate with regard to pathologic first-ray hypermobility and its role in hallux valgus deformity and correction. We present a discussion on the use of proximal first-ray osteotomies in the surgical treatment for hallux valgus as a valid option compared with first-tarsometatarsal arthrodesis.
- Recent and historical literature tells us that stability of the first ray is a function of the alignment and reestablishment of retrograde stabilizing forces at the first tarsometatarsal joint.

Both podiatric and orthopedic surgeons treat hallux valgus. Approximately 33% of individuals in shod populations have some degree of hallux valgus[1] and more than 200,000 hallux valgus operations are performed in the United States each year.[2] The deformity itself varies from mild to severe (**Fig. 1**). The literature describes numerous operative procedures for this common malady. The etiology and best operative treatment, however, remain controversial. This article first reviews the utility of first-metatarsal osteotomies in the correction of hallux valgus or metatarsus primus varus (MPV), and then demonstrates the effectiveness of first-metatarsal osteotomies in restoring stable mechanics of the first ray without the need for arthrodesis.

Many reports in the literature suggest the Lapidus procedure, or first-tarsometatarsal fusion, is the only procedure to adequately address bunion with a moderate or larger intermetatarsal angle secondary to the "atavistic" relationship

Disclosures: Dr Sorensen – Consultant and Design Surgeon for Stryker Orthopedics and Treace Medical; Dr Cottom – Consultant/Design Surgeon for Arthrex and Consultant for Stryker/SBi.
[a] Weil Foot & Ankle Institute, Golf River Professional Building, 1455 East Golf Road, Des Plaines, IL 60016, USA; [b] Coastal Orthopedics and Sports Medicine, Bradenton, FL, USA
* Corresponding author.
E-mail address: mdsoren34@gmail.com

Clin Podiatr Med Surg 32 (2015) 355–374
http://dx.doi.org/10.1016/j.cpm.2015.03.009
0891-8422/15/$ – see front matter © 2015 Elsevier Inc. All rights reserved.

podiatric.theclinics.com

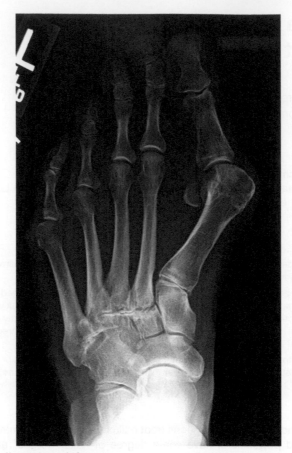

Fig. 1. Severe hallux valgus deformity.

between first-ray hypermobility and hallux valgus formation. Proximal metatarsal osteotomies are often indicated for mild, moderate, and severe hallux valgus deformities. Several recent published studies have suggested that realignment of the first ray through osteotomy in the appropriately selected patient may negate the need for first-metatarsal–cuneiform fusion. Hypermobility or instability of the first ray often can be adequately stabilized by realignment of the bone and soft tissue structures. This allows the effects of the windlass mechanism of the plantar fascia, as well as the stabilizing force of the peroneus longus, to be reestablished without sacrifice of the first tarsometatarsal joint (TMTJ).

HISTORY

Surgical intervention for hallux valgus dates back at least to Gernet in 1836. Nineteenth-century physicians surmised the notion of structural change for hallux valgus. Their efforts led to the introduction of the Reverdin osteotomy[3] in 1881 and to others, such as the Mayo,[4] the Keller,[5] and the Brandes.[6]

The evolution of modern-day operative treatment for hallux valgus has journeyed through innumerable biomechanical, genetic, traumatic, and idiopathic etiologic theories. It seems in recent years, the gestalt of surgical intervention of hallux valgus has teetered between 2 dominating theories, one based on biomechanics and the other based on clinical study. Without a single unifying theory on which to base surgical intervention, foot and ankle surgeons have formed their own opinions regarding their procedure selection and ideology.

The active debate centers at first metatarsocuneiform joint fusion versus metatarsal osteotomy for surgical intervention of hallux valgus and stabilization of the first ray. Each camp has sound biomechanical, theoretic, and clinical research to support one over the other. This article examines the argument for osteotomy with distal soft tissue release (DSTR).

INDICATIONS

Indications for surgical intervention include a symptomatic clinical and radiographic hallux valgus deformity. Before surgical intervention, exhaustion of conservation care is recommended, including, but not limited to, ice, rest, accommodative padding, nonsteroidal anti-inflammatory drug therapy, orthoses, splinting, physical therapy, and shoe-gear modification. On failure of conservative measures, surgical intervention can be considered in the appropriately selected patient.

Comorbidities, such as diabetes mellitus, rheumatoid arthritis, peripheral neuropathy, tobacco or drug abuse, and history of blood clot or hematologic disorder, among others, need to be carefully considered. Also, the social support structure and work environment are important considerations when making the decision for or against surgical intervention. The patient should clearly understand the postoperative course, expected outcomes, and potential complications and risks before going forward.

PROCEDURE SELECTION

There is a general consensus that many factors figure into the selection of corrective surgery for a particular bunion deformity. This decision is partly based on the degree and severity of deformity, the involvement of soft tissue and bone malalignment, and the surgeon's expertise and comfort with certain procedures. Most surgeons agree that for a "mild" deformity, a distal osteotomy is appropriate and provides reliable correction. It is in cases of moderate to severe deformity that surgeons seem to have varied opinions about procedures involving osteotomies of the diaphysis or base of the first metatarsal. The necessity of moving the correction more proximal is based on the simple mathematical/physical understanding of deformity.

DISTAL OSTEOTOMIES

Distal osteotomy in the treatment of hallux valgus deformity is generally reserved for first-second intermetatarsal angles of lesser magnitude with the upper limit generally noted at 14° to 15°. Originators of distal osteotomies have recommended no more than 25% to 50% translation of the distal fragment in relation to the metatarsal shaft.[7–12] Geometric and physical analysis has shown that the 25% to 50% magnitude of capital fragment lateral displacement lacks the ability to correct moderate to large first-second intermetatarsal angles.[13–16]

Other factors to consider in the decision for distal osteotomy correction include the presence of metatarsus adductus or skewfoot deformity (**Fig. 2**), as well as any hindfoot valgus deformity, which places the apex of the deformity much farther proximal and may render a distal osteotomy inadequate.

Following reports by Austin and colleagues,[7,17] the chevron osteotomy has become widely accepted for the correction of mild to moderate hallux valgus deformity. The

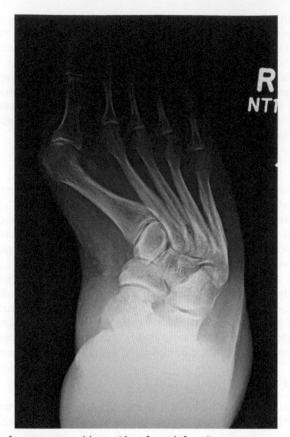

Fig. 2. Example of metatarsus adductus/skewfoot deformity.

"V" shape of the osteotomy is thought to provide inherent stability with the ability of the capital fragment to impact on the shaft of the metatarsal after translation. This quality aides in the strength of the construct. In fact, some purport the lack in need for fixation due to this stability. That being said, subsequent investigators have noted more loss of correction or avascular necrosis in chevron bunionectomies performed without fixation.[15,18] Muhlbauer[19] performed a prospective study using Kirschner-wire (k-wire) fixation for the chevron bunionectomy in 55 feet. At an average follow-up of 34 months, there was no case of metatarsal head displacement or loss of correction. Foot and ankle surgeons today generally favor the use of fixation as an aid for stability and report overall satisfaction among patients and surgeons with the procedure (**Fig. 3**). The distal chevron osteotomy is generally reserved for cases of mild to moderate deformity; however, there have been recent studies that suggest that this procedure provides an effective and reliable means of correcting hallux valgus regardless of severity of deformity.[20,21]

Generally, the procedure can be performed on an outpatient basis under local/minimal anesthetic concentration anesthesia, with or without a tourniquet. Per surgeon preference, the patient can be casted or placed into a soft dressing with stiff-soled walking shoe. One of the "selling points" of a distal procedure is the ability to maintain the patient on partial weight-bearing immediately after surgical intervention with weight placed back on the heel until adequate bone healing is noted on radiographs.

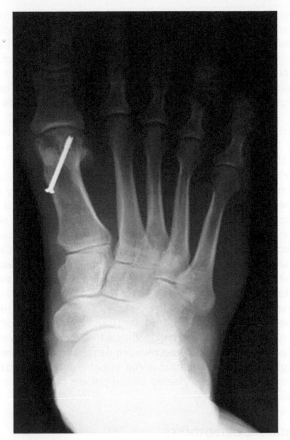

Fig. 3. Distal chevron bunionectomy.

Early weight-bearing decreases the morbidity, overall recovery time, and chances of deep vein thrombosis. Patients also appreciate the freedom weight-bearing mobility offers them.

As stated, the distal osteotomies have a role in mild deformity correction but are limited because they are distal. The lever arm in correction is short and thus limited to the lesser deformity. As the point of deformity correction moves more proximal, larger degrees of deformity can be addressed.

MIDSHAFT OSTEOTOMY

Virtually any metatarsal osteotomy can be performed in the diaphyseal shaft and subsequently retain the label of midshaft osteotomy. The scarf osteotomy and the "long-arm" chevron osteotomy have gained popularity in recent years secondary to their inherent stability. Weil[22] and Zygmont and colleagues[23] began to popularize the scarf in the early 1980s, and Barouk[24] took the osteotomy to Europe in the early 1990s. A number of modifications to the scarf have been described, including the short scarf, the long scarf, and the inverted scarf.[24–27]

The scarf bunionectomy is a tricut osteotomy that can be used to correct intermetatarsal angles from 12° to 23°, abnormal proximal articular set angle values up to 10°, and plantar or dorsal displaced metatarsals, making it a utilitarian procedure.[22,28–30] The interlocking scarf has been used for centuries as a carpentry principle. Its primary contribution is its inherent stability and ability to distribute load. The inherent stability of the scarf bunionectomy allows concurrent bilateral correction, immediate postoperative weight-bearing in a surgical shoe without crutches, return to athletic shoes, and the beginning of physical therapy at 1 week after surgery.[31] The osteotomy is amenable to single-screw or multiscrew fixation; however, 2 points of fixation are preferred.[28]

Two-plane correction can be obtained with the scarf during lateral translation of the capital fragment by orienting the horizontal cut plantarly or dorsally. In addition, lengthening and shortening of the metatarsal can be achieved using the scarf.[32,33]

However, reports have indicated that the scarf is not without complications.[34,35] The troughing phenomenon is more frequent in the short scarf secondary to the proximal arm location in the less-compact diaphyseal medullary bone, while the distal segment remains in the more compact metaphyseal metatarsal head. This is reportedly more limited in the long scarf, as both arms are located within metaphyseal bone.[22] The distal and proximal vertical arms of the osteotomy should be limited to 2 to 3 mm in depth to avoid the stress riser into the dorsal/plantar cortex and to decrease the incidence and magnitude of "troughing."[32] Performing the distal cut in the metaphyseal region of the metatarsal will aid in prevention of troughing, whereas keeping the longitudinal cut in the plantar one-third of the metatarsal will prevent stress riser.[28]

In a study by Saxena and St Louis[36] comparing the corrective capacities of the distal extended chevron versus the scarf in hallux valgus treatment, the investigators found the scarf and extended chevron osteotomies are capable of adequately reducing the hallux valgus angle and intermetatarsal angle in patients with moderate to severe hallux valgus. These 2 techniques yielded similar patient outcomes in terms of stiffness, pain, and satisfaction.

PROXIMAL METATARSAL OSTEOTOMIES

As a general principle, the severity of the hallux valgus deformity dictates treatment options. The need for metatarsal base osteotomies arises on encountering patients with first-second intermetatarsal angles of greater magnitude, with the spectrum threshold of approximately 13° to 15° and greater.[37] The available degree of correction in the proximal osteotomy is substantially greater than that for distal or midshaft osteotomies, given the more proximal location of the axis of rotation.

In the early twentieth century, Loison and others[38–40] reported on their experience with proximal osteotomies. Several proximal osteotomies have been reported to yield good clinical results, including osteotomies involving the proximal chevron, closing and opening base wedges, the Ludloff procedure, the crescentic procedure, and the Mau procedure.[37,41–51]

The proximal crescentic procedure, as popularized by Mann and colleagues,[47] is the only osteotomy of this kind that requires a crescentic saw blade. The proposed benefits include a truly rotational osteotomy with ability to correct in all 3 planes with minimal shortening. The long-standing concerns, however, are its inherent lack of stability and subsequent complication of dorsiflexion malunion, as well as difficulty in fixation.[43,47,51–53]

Several studies have compared the crescentic to other proximal osteotomies. A prospective randomized comparison (level II evidence) of the proximal crescentic versus the proximal chevron denoted favorable radiographic correction and clinical outcomes for both. However, dorsiflexion malunion was observed in 17% of the proximal crescentic osteotomies (**Fig. 4**).[54]

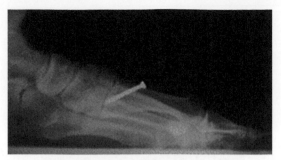

Fig. 4. Proximal crescentic bunionectomy showing dorsal malunion.

A level II evidentiary study by Hyer and colleagues[55] compared the crescentic and Mau osteotomies. Satisfactory correction was noted in both groups and no statistical difference was seen in the magnitude of correction between the two. Statistical differences were noted between the crescentic and Mau with regard to complications. Transarticular hardware positioned in the first TMTJ occurred in 40% of crescentic osteotomy cases. The nonunion rate was 50% in the crescentic group and only 4.2% in the Mau group. The investigators did relate, however, that given a longer period for follow-up, the union rate may have increased for the crescentic. They concluded that given the amount of correction achieved using the Mau, and its lower incidence of postoperative complications, they prefer it to the crescentic for correction of moderate to severe hallux valgus.

In one of the original articles describing the procedure, Mann and colleagues[47] noted dorsiflexion malunions in 28% of cases. Numerous investigators have made modifications to the crescentic in attempts to aid overall stability. Jones and colleagues[54] described a technique orienting the saw blade correctly in the coronal plane to minimize the risk of initial dorsiflexion malpositioning. Perhaps the most logical modification to the crescentic osteotomy itself was the one suggested by Cohen and colleagues.[56] This modification uses a plantar shelf exiting distal to the osteotomy, thus imparting more stability to the cut as well as ease of fixation.

The advent of foot-specific locked plating may lead to decreased incidence of dorsal malunion for all proximal osteotomies, including that seen in the crescentic. A study by Gallentine and colleagues[57] concluded a locked plate construct held alignment and position of the proximal chevron first-ray osteotomy without clinical evidence of transfer lesion or hardware-related symptoms. In the authors' recent experience, locked plating has greatly facilitated success toward correction with the crescentic osteotomy. The robust nature of the locked plating systems largely eliminates the incidence of dorsal malunion or any instability secondary to the inherence of the osteotomy construct. Also, by eliminating the need for interfragmentary screw placement, locked plating diminishes the possibility of inadvertent intra-articular screw placement. In context, however, again because of the disarticulated and unstable nature of this bone cut, a significant degree of difficulty in initial correction on the table can be encountered with the crescentic.

The Mau osteotomy of the proximal first metatarsal is another procedure used for the correction of moderate to severe hallux valgus (**Fig. 5**). It entails the use of a through-and-through, transverse plane osteotomy that extends plantar-proximal to dorsal-distal and has been referred to as a reverse Ludloff osteotomy.[49,50] It has triplanar correction capacity. Mau, it is said, questioned the stability of the Ludloff

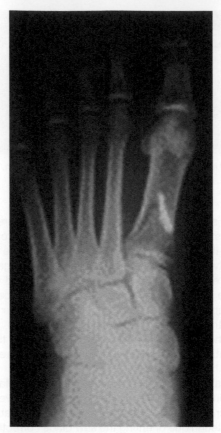

Fig. 5. Mau osteotomy for bunion correction.

osteotomy and used the dorsal shelf to resist the potentially disruptive forces of weight-bearing.[50] Although early use of both the Ludloff and Mau osteotomies did not involve internal fixation, more recent reports of these procedures describe the use of osteosynthesis techniques to minimize the risk of complication related to bone healing.[50,58] Moreover, the Mau osteotomy, because of the presence of a dorsal shelf to resist dorsal displacement forces, may impart superior intrinsic stability in comparison with other proximal osteotomies.[55]

In an evaluation of the relative fatigue strength (load to failure) of the Mau, Ludloff, and crescentic osteotomies, Acevedo and colleagues[59] reported that the Mau and Ludloff osteotomies, in comparison with the crescentic osteotomy, were more resistant to fatigue failure. In a comparison of 6 cadaveric first-metatarsal shaft osteotomies, the Mau osteotomy was shown to be statistically significantly superior in strength and stiffness compared with all other osteotomies except the Ludloff.[58]

The Ludloff osteotomy was introduced in 1913 but failed to gain acceptance because the original description did not include fixation.[60] The advent of screw fixation brought about new interest in the procedure.[45] The Ludloff osteotomy is oriented from proximal-dorsal to distal-plantar and can be oriented in the sagittal plane so as to influence dorsiflexion or plantarflexion on translation/rotation in the transverse plane, thus allowing correction in all 3 planes. On fixation, the first screw is placed before the osteotomy is completed, allowing the surgeon to maintain full control of the osteotomy throughout the procedure.[45] In a recent study of 110 feet, Saxena and St Louis[36] demonstrated favorable results performing the Ludloff osteotomy with medial locking plate fixation.

A number of recent clinical series (level IV evidence) have analyzed the modified Ludloff in combination with a distal soft tissue procedure. Trnka and colleagues[61] related favorable outcome results on the largest cohort of patients known to date having undergone the Ludloff. The mean American Orthopedic Foot and Ankle Score (AOFAS) improved to 88 points from 53 points at 34-month follow-up. The mean hallux valgus angle decreased significantly from 35° preoperatively to 9° at the most recent follow-up, and the mean intermetatarsal angle decreased significantly to 8° from 17°. All osteotomy sites united without dorsiflexion malunion, but did have a mean first-metatarsal shortening of 2.2 mm.

The authors would also assert that the Mau and Ludloff osteotomies are less difficult to perform and can be learned more quickly than the crescentic osteotomy. This makes for fewer inadvertent or operator-related postoperative sequelae.

The opening wedge proximal metatarsal osteotomy, initially described by Trethowan[40] in 1923, did not gain early acceptance because of lack of adequate fixation and corrective maintenance. With the advent of fixed-angle wedge plates and locked plating, the procedure has become more viable in recent years (**Fig. 6**). Bone graft

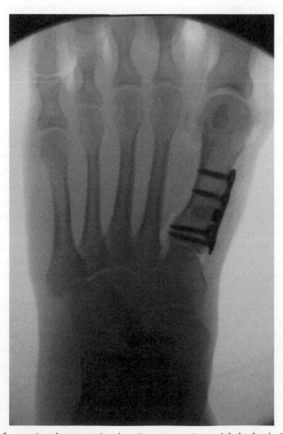

Fig. 6. Example of opening base wedge bunion correction with locked plate fixation.

(autograft, allograft, or bone substitute) is generally required to fill the gap left by the opening wedge. The benefit of the opening wedge is maintenance of length, which can be necessary in those patients with a short first metatarsal. There has been, to date, no evidence demonstrating that the opening wedge elongates the metatarsal. In addition, this osteotomy can also correct deformity in 3 planes by orienting the axis/hinge of the osteotomy in the coronal and sagittal planes.

The closing base wedge osteotomy is similar to the opening wedge osteotomy. However, with the closing base wedge osteotomy, the hinge is maintained on the medial metatarsal cortex and a wedge of bone removed. Reports have described the wedge being removed in an orientation perpendicular to the metatarsal long axis as well as oblique to the metatarsal long axis. The oblique closing wedge is more amenable to 2-screw fixation. Also, because the apex/hinge is theoretically stronger when placed in the proximal medial-most corner of the first metatarsal, an oblique closing wedge is theoretically more stable. Skepticism has been encountered with this osteotomy based on reports of dorsiflexion malunion, as well as "shortening."[62–64] Also, with orientation of the axis and the triplanar correction capacity of the closing wedge, plantarflexion or dorsiflexion can be "built in" to the osteotomy so as to further stabilize the forefoot on correction.

The proximal chevron osteotomy without modification is purely translational. Subsequently correction capacity is based on the width of the proximal metatarsal shaft. Sammarco and colleagues[65–67] modified the chevron by incorporating an opening wedge principle for his base procedure, therefore adding the rotational component to the correction. The large contact area allows for adequate screw or plate fixation or combination with k-wire. A level II investigation comparing the proximal chevron to the crescentic denoted adequate correction for both, but a significant difference in dorsiflexion malunion between the two with a 0% incidence for the chevron versus 17% incidence for the crescentic.[54]

LAPIDUS

First tarso-metatarsal arthrodesis was first described by Albrecht in 1911.[68] Paul Lapidus subsequently described the procedure in 1934 for correction of MPV deformity and from there it has gained notoriety.[69] The indications are an MPV deformity that presents with a high first and second intermetatarsal angle, a hypermobile first ray, as well as recurrent MPV deformity. Advantages of the Lapidus include correction of the deformity at the apex as well as the ability to stabilize the medial column of the foot.[69,70] Concerns over the procedure traditionally stem from increased nonunion rates as well as prolonged periods of non–weight-bearing.[71] Since Lapidus' description, many fixation constructs have been described. The use of k-wires, staples, compression screws, plate fixation, external fixation, and combinations of the different methods have all been advocated.[72]

With any arthrodesis procedure, nonunion can result and arthrodesis of the first TMTJ is no exception. Nonunion of the first TMTJ has been reported to be as high as 25%.[73] Recent advances in surgical technique along with rigid internal fixation have improved the rates of nonunion substantially with a range between 2% and 12%, respectively.[72–76] In a retrospective study by Patel and colleagues,[75] 227 Lapidus procedures were studied and the nonunion rate was found to be 5.3%. Furthermore, Scranton and colleagues[77] reported a nonunion rate of 2% in their study of 88 patients with a plantar interfragmentary screw and medial locking plate construct.

Sangeorzan and Hansen[71] introduced crossed screws in 1989 and this fixation technique has been widely accepted. Biomechanical studies remain controversial in the literature. A study by Gruber and colleagues[74] found that 2 crossed screws were equal in rigidity when compared with 2 crossed screws along with a dorsomedial plate. Scranton and colleagues[77] carried out a cadaveric biomechanical study comparing 2 crossed 4.0 screws versus a locking compression plate with an intraplate compression screw.[77] The ultimate load to failure was 78 N in the crossing screw group and 108 N in the locking plate compression screw construct. Cottom and Rigby[78] performed a biomechanical study comparing a compression plate with an intraplate compression screw to the same compression plate along with a plantar interfragmentary compression screw on the tension side of the fusion site. They found that with the addition of the plantar screw, the load-to-failure rate increased from 205.5 N to 383.2 N, respectively.

Return to weight-bearing after the Lapidus procedure is varied. The risk of nonunion has forced surgeons to implement a prolonged non–weight-bearing course for these patients.[79] Immobilizing patients for 6 to 8 weeks can lead to muscle atrophy, deep vein thrombosis, osteopenia, and pulmonary embolism.[80] The disadvantages of non–weight-bearing along with the advent of more rigid fixation constructs have allowed surgeons to reduce the period non–weight-bearing with some advocating for immediate weight-bearing.[73,79,81,82] The decision on weight-bearing status is multifactorial and should be individualized on each patient according the presence or absence of comorbidities and the patient's general health. Sangeorzan and Hansen[71] allowed early weight-bearing with crossed screws and reported a 92% union rate. Sorensen and colleagues[82] advocated weight-bearing at 2 weeks when a medial locking plate was used with 100% union rate.

The authors' current preferred method includes the use of 1 or 2 compression screws crossing the first TMTJ, followed by a locked plate placed medially to engage the strongest inherent construct against cantilever/bending forces through the midfoot on ambulation (**Fig. 7**). Lapidus for the correction of MPV is a powerful procedure. Large intermetatarsal angles can be corrected at the apex of the deformity along with stabilization of the medial column. New advances in techniques and fixation

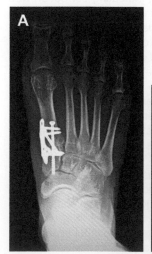
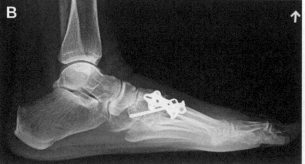

Fig. 7. Example of Lapidus bunionectomy with fixation, anteroposterior (A) and Lateral (B) views.

constructs have significantly decreased nonunion rates and have allowed foot and ankle surgeons to successfully institute early weight-bearing protocols for this procedure.

OSTEOTOMY VERSUS ARTHRODESIS

The debate about whether or not to perform a Lapidus has to do with the biomechanical domain of hallux valgus. The individual ideology of each surgeon drives the choice of metatarsal base osteotomy versus fusion. However, depending on the case, Lapidus fusion and the proximal metatarsal osteotomy each has a role in hallux valgus correction. The key in this decision is to differentiate a case of a truly unstable first ray or medial column from a case of a hypermobile first ray secondary to development of hallux valgus. Determining this assertive differentiation is beyond the scope of this article; however, we review the biomechanical supporting arguments for the metatarsal basilar osteotomies, and assert that, at times, it is this chicken before that egg. In addition, it is the authors' belief, supported by a significant volume of evidence-based literature, that not every case of hallux valgus is hypermobile.

Morton,[83] in 1928, first introduced the theory of first-ray hypermobility. The causative connection between first-ray hypermobility and hallux valgus deformity was then asserted by Lapidus.[84,85] Contrary to widespread belief, neither investigator quantified hypermobility.[86] Klaue and colleagues[87] designed an external caliper for the measurement of first-ray mobility, and this was later validated by Jones and colleagues.[88] Klaue and colleagues[87] and Jones and colleagues[88] further defined the first ray as hypermobile if there were 9 mm or more of sagittal motion as measured with this device.

Others have shown an association between hallux valgus and an increased mobility of the first ray.[89–91] The numeric value or quantity of first-ray mobility had not been reported preoperatively or postoperatively in these studies, even amidst contention that a hypermobile first ray is indication enough for a first-metatarsal–cuneiform fusion.[86] In studies by Dreeben and Mann[92] and by Veri and colleagues,[93] DSTR and proximal first-metatarsal osteotomy for treatment of hallux valgus had low recurrence rates at both intermediate and long-term follow-up, indicating correction was maintained despite failure to fuse the first-tarsometatarsal articulation.

In a recent cadaver study of specimens with hallux valgus deformity, a 50% reduction in sagittal plane mobility (to 5.2 mm from 11.0 mm) was observed following a distal soft tissue realignment DSTR and proximal first-metatarsal osteotomy.[94] Additionally, a recent prospective clinical study of 108 patients with hallux valgus and MPV was published.[86] Increased preoperative mobility of the first ray was regularly and consistently reduced to a normal range following proximal crescentic osteotomy and DSTR and without fusion of the first TMTJ.[86] These studies further suggest that realignment of the first ray and reorientation of the soft tissue support structures, whether by soft tissue releases/transfers and osteotomies or by first-tarsometatarsal fusion is the crucial step in MPV and hallux valgus correction.

The corrective power of first-ray realignment and soft tissue balancing is demonstrated time and again in the rheumatoid foot reconstruction. Frequently, in addition to severe hallux valgus and lesser metatarsophalangeal joint dislocations, there is proximal first-tarsometatarsal instability demonstrated on radiograph (**Fig. 8**). Once the soft tissues are rebalanced and the first ray realigned, the proximal instability is reduced and stabilized (**Fig. 9**) without the need of proximal joint arthrodesis.

Another study by Kim and colleagues,[95] of 82 proximal chevron osteotomies and DSTR for symptomatic hallux valgus, showed clinical dorsiflexion mobility of the first

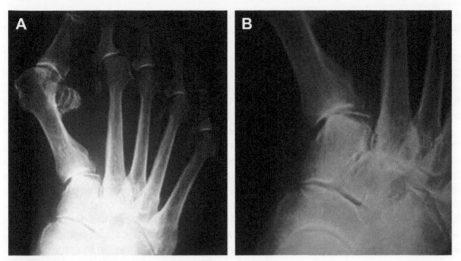

Fig. 8. First tarsometatarsal joint instability.

ray to be reduced with clinical significance at an average of 1-year postoperative follow-up. They concluded that, secondary to stability of the first ray imparted by correction of the realignment metatarsal base osteotomy and DSTR, the surgical indication for the proximal osteotomy procedure can be recommended more broadly to include the correction of hallux valgus deformity accompanying first-ray hypermobility

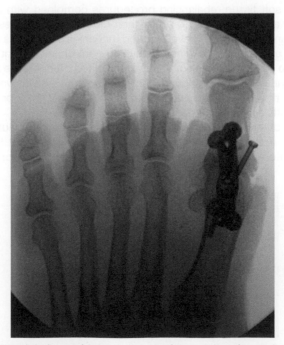

Fig. 9. First metatarsalphalangeal joint fusion used to stabilize the medial column.

instead of the Lapidus procedure, which has more complications and a lower satisfaction rate.

These studies and many more suggest a stabilizing effect created by realignment of bone and soft tissue structures along the first-ray axis. There is a retrograde loading phenomenon that is reestablished back into the first TMTJ, thus reducing the degree of preoperative "hypermobility." The stabilizing forces of the windlass mechanism of the plantar fascia, as well as the pull of the peroneus longus tendon at the first-metatarsal base, are thought to be keys in first-ray stability without fusion.

Moving forward, one parameter proposed to assess sagittal plane instability at the first tarsometatarsal is the metatarsal-medial cuneiform angle or plantar gapping/wedging seen on the lateral weight-bearing foot radiograph.[96] It has not, however, been assessed in relationship to actual quantified mobility of the first ray.[86] In the recent Coughlin and Jones study,[86] 23% of the feet demonstrated preoperative plantar gapping on radiograph (**Fig. 10**). Those with gapping had, on average, a significantly greater hallux valgus deformity than those without preoperative gapping. There was, however, no significant difference between those with and those without preoperative plantar gapping with respect to the mobility of the first ray. In the study group, the gapping resolved after realignment of the first ray in one-third of the feet. There was no difference in the mean preoperative hallux valgus angle between the feet with residual gapping and those in which the gapping resolved. The group with residual gapping tended to have a larger angular correction compared with those in which gapping resolved. The mean mobility of the first ray was slightly higher both preoperatively and postoperatively in the group in which gapping resolved. Again, the findings of this study suggest a stabilizing effect is created by successfully realigning the first-ray axis by, in this case, proximal metatarsal osteotomy. These studies strongly suggest stability of the first ray can be achieved successfully and correction can be maintained when the imbalances of bone and soft tissue are corrected. This may be done with distal soft tissue rebalancing procedures combined with proximal metatarsal osteotomy and not necessarily a first-tarsometatarsal arthrodesis.

Meanwhile, many investigators have asserted that ankle equinus, as well as pes planus deformity, is also associated with the development of hallux valgus.[97–99] In more recent studies, no correlation was noted between limited preoperative ankle dorsiflexion and the magnitude of the preoperative or postoperative hallux valgus deformity, the magnitude of the angular correction, the postoperative AOFAS, or the postoperative subjective satisfaction of the patient.[86]

Sarrafian and others[90,100,101] have identified the plantar aponeurosis as a key component of first-ray stability. Coughlin and Jones[86] suggest that the realignment of the first ray restores the normal anatomic relationships and function of the intrinsic

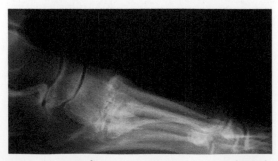

Fig. 10. Plantar gapping shown at first tarsometatarsal joint on lateral view.

muscles, the extrinsic muscles, and the plantar aponeurosis, and that this leads to a reduction in first-ray mobility. It is thought that the stability of the first ray is a function of the alignment of the first ray and is not an intrinsic characteristic of the first meta-tarsocuneiform joint. This really is the crux in on-going discussions regarding the nature and appropriateness of the proximal first-metatarsal osteotomy in conjunction with DSTR for treatment of hallux valgus deformity.

In a recent forum, Drs Donald Green and Peter Kim[102] eloquently describe their approach to hallux valgus. They state the obvious advantage to the metatarsal basilar osteotomy as allowing for continued natural range of motion throughout the rest of the joints in the foot. They further describe the foot's "tensegrity" as part of an integrated truss system in which there are only tension and compression elements rather than levers or bending moments and without any torque at the joints.[103] This creates a me-chanically efficient system that stores and returns energy with smooth motion in an efficient gait pattern with muscles developing tension on the fascia to provide protec-tion, energy return, and smooth motion.[102] They further relate that arthrodesis leads to disintegration of gait with increased energy consumption, decreased gait speed, and increased pressure on other joints. They point to the example of ankle arthrodesis and its sequelae on adjacent joint health.

SUMMARY

These arguments and review of the literature are not meant to suggest the Lapidus arthrodesis has no role in hallux valgus correction or first-ray stabilization. This proce-dure can be used effectively and efficiently for both. This discussion is meant to simply point out that proximal osteotomies and soft tissue rebalancing also can successfully accomplish these goals. Each case of hallux valgus is different and has a unique etiology. A procedure should be selected only after this etiology is properly identified and evalu-ated. The quest for definitive, irrefutable etiologic definition of the common hallux valgus foot deformity continues. To date, no all-encompassing theory or clinically proven entity has emerged to settle the debate with regard to pathologic first-ray hypermobility and its role in hallux valgus deformity and correction. We present a discussion on the use of proximal first-ray osteotomies in the surgical treatment for hallux valgus as a valid option compared with first-tarsometatarsal arthrodesis. Recent and historical literature tells us that stability of the first ray is a function of the alignment and reestablishment of retro-grade stabilizing forces at the first TMTJ. This realignment and stabilization may be accomplished with the use of distal soft tissue and proximal osteotomy procedures.

REFERENCES

1. Sim Fook L, Hodgson AR. A comparison of foot forms among the non-shoe and shoe-wearing Chinese population. J Bone Joint Surg Am 1958;40-A:1058–62.
2. Coughlin MJ, Thompson FM. The high price of high fashion footwear. Instr Course Lect 1995;44:371–7.
3. Reverdin J. De la deviation en dehors du gros orl (hallux valgus) et son traite-ment chirurgical. Trans Int Med Congress 1881;2:408–12 [in French].
4. Mayo CH. The surgical treatment of bunion. Ann Surg 1908;48:300–2.
5. Keller WL. The surgical treatment of bunions and hallux valgus. NY Med 1904; 80:741–2.
6. Brandes M. Zur operation therapie des hallux valgus. [For the surgical therapy of hallux valgus]. Zentralbl Chir 1924;56:243–4 [in German].
7. Austin DW, Leventen EO. A new osteotomy for hallux valgus. Clin Orthop 1981; 157:25–30.

8. Corless JR. A modification of the Mitchell procedure. J Bone Joint Surg 1976; 58-B:128–32.
9. Johnson KA, Cofield RH, Morrey BF. Chevron osteotomy for hallux valgus. Clin Orthop 1979;142:44–7.
10. Mann RA, Coughlin MJ. Adult hallux valgus. In: Coughlin MJ, Mann RA, editors. Surgery of the foot and ankle. 7th edition. St Louis (MO): Mosby; 1999. p. 150–269.
11. Myerson MS. Hallux valgus. In: Meyerson MS, editor. Foot and ankle disorders. Philadelphia: Saunders; 2000. p. 213–88.
12. Richardson EG, Donley BG. Disorders of hallux. In: Canle ST, editor. Campbell's operative orthopaedics. 10th edition. Philadelphia: Mosby; 2003. p. 3915–4015.
13. Badwey TM, Dutkowsky JP, Graves SC, et al. An anatomical basis for the degree of displacement of the distal chevron osteotomy in the treatment of hallux valgus. Foot Ankle Int 1997;18:213–5.
14. Harper MC. Correction of metatarsus primus varus with the chevron metatarsal osteotomy. Clin Orthop 1989;243:180–3.
15. Jahss MH, Troy AI, Kummer F. Roentgenographic and mathematical analysis of first metatarsal osteotomies for metatarsus primus varus: a comparative study. Foot Ankle Int 1985;5:280–321.
16. Sarrafian SK. A method of predicting the degree of functional correction of the metatarsus primus varus with a distal lateral displacement osteotomy in hallux valgus. Foot Ankle Int 1985;5:322–6.
17. Miller S, Croce WA. The Austin procedure for surgical correction of hallux abducto valgus deformity. J Am Podiatry Assoc 1979;69:110–8.
18. Hattrup SJ, Johnson KA. Chevron osteotomy: analysis of factors in patients' dissatisfaction. Foot Ankle 1985;5:327–32.
19. Muhlbauer M, Zembsch A, Trnka HJ. Kurzfristige ergebnisse der modifizierten chevron-osteotomie mit weichteiltechnik und bohrdrahtfixation—eine prospective studie. [Short-term results of modified chevron osteotomy with soft tissue technique and guide wire fixation—a prospective study]. Z Orthop Ihre Grenzgeb 2001;139:435–9 [in German].
20. Moon JY, Lee KB, Seon JK, et al. Outcomes of proximal chevron osteotomy for moderate versus severe hallux valgus deformities. Foot Ankle Int 2012;33(8): 637–43.
21. Bai LB, Lee KB, Seo CY, et al. Distal chevron osteotomy with distal soft tissue procedure for moderate to severe hallux valgus deformity. Foot Ankle Int 2010;31(8):683–8.
22. Weil LS. Scarf osteotomy for correction of hallux valgus. Historical perspective, surgical technique, and results. Foot Ankle Clin 2000;5(3):559–80.
23. Zygmont KH, Gudas CJ, Laros GS. Bunionectomy with intertarsal screw fixation. J Am Podiatr Med Assoc 1989;79:322–9.
24. Barouk LS. Scarf osteotomy for hallux valgus correction. Local anatomy, surgical technique, and combination with other forefoot procedures. Foot Ankle Clin 2000;5(3):525–58.
25. Pollack RA, Bellacosa RA, Higgins KR, et al. Critical evaluation of the short "Z" bunionectomy. J Foot Surg 1989;28:158–61.
26. Barouk LS. Osteotomies of the great toe. J Foot Surg 1992;31:388–99.
27. Kristen KH, Berger C, Stelzig S, et al. The SCARF osteotomy for the correction of hallux valgus deformities. Foot Ankle Int 2002;23:221–9.
28. Weil L Jr, Bowen M. Scarf osteotomy for correction of hallux abducto valgus deformity. Clin Podiatr Med Surg 2014;31(2):233–46.

29. Weil L Jr. Mastering the scarf procedure for hallux valgus correction. Foot Ankle Spec 2009;2(3):151–5.
30. Barouk LS. Scarf osteotomy of the first metatarsal in the treatment of hallux valgus. Foot Dis 1995;2:35–48.
31. Fridman R, Cain JD, Weil LJ, et al. Unilateral versus bilateral first ray surgery: a prospective study of 186 consecutive cases–patient satisfaction, cost to society, and complications. Foot Ankle Spec 2009;2:123–9.
32. Coetzee JC, Rippstein P. Surgical strategies: scarf osteotomy for hallux valgus. Foot Ankle Int 2007;28(4):529–35.
33. Deenik AR, Pilot P, Brandt SE, et al. Scarf versus chevron osteotomy in hallux valgus: a randomized controlled trial in 96 patients. Foot Ankle Int 2007;28(5): 537–41.
34. Coetzee JC. Scarf osteotomy for hallux valgus correction: the dark side. Foot Ankle Int 2003;24:29–33.
35. Trnka HJ. Osteotomies for hallux valgus correction. Foot Ankle Clin 2005;10: 15–33.
36. Saxena A, St Louis M. Medial locking plate versus screw fixation for fixation of the Ludloff osteotomy. J Foot Ankle Surg 2013;52(2):153–7.
37. Pehlivan O, Akmaz I, Solakoglu C, et al. Proximal oblique crescentic osteotomy in hallux valgus. J Am Podiatr Med Assoc 2004;94(1):43–6.
38. Loison M. Note sure letraitment chirurgical du hallux valgus d'apres l'etude radiographique de la deformation. Bull Soc Chir Paris 1901;27:528–31 [in French].
39. Balacescu J. Un caz de hallux valgus simetric. Rev Chir 1903;7:128–35.
40. Trethowan J. Hallux valgus. In: Choyce CC, editor. A system of surgery. New York: Hoeber, PG; 1923. p. 1046–9.
41. McClusky LC, Johnson JE, Wynarsky GT, et al. Comparison of stability of proximal crescentic metatarsal osteotomy and proximal horizontal "V" osteotomy. Foot Ankle Int 1994;15(5):263–70.
42. Easley ME, Kiebzak GM, Davis WH, et al. Prospective, randomized comparison of proximal crescentic and proximal chevron osteotomies for correction of hallux valgus deformity. Foot Ankle Int 1996;17(6):307–16.
43. Markbreiter LA, Thompson FM. Proximal metatarsal osteotomy in hallux valgus correction: a comparison of crescentic and chevron procedures. Foot Ankle Int 1997;18(2):71–6.
44. Vora AM, Myerson MS. First metatarsal osteotomy nonunion and malunion. Foot Ankle Clin 2005;10(1):35–54.
45. Chiodo CP, Schon LC, Myerson MS. Clinical results with the Ludloff osteotomy for correction of adult hallux valgus. Foot Ankle Int 2004;25(8):532–6.
46. Saxena A, McCammon D. The Ludloff osteotomy: a critical analysis. J Foot Ankle Surg 1997;36(2):100–5.
47. Mann RA, Rudicel S, Graves SC. Repair of hallux valgus with a distal soft-tissue procedure and proximal metatarsal osteotomy. A long-term follow-up. J Bone Joint Surg Am 1992;74(1):124–9.
48. Thorardson DB, Leventen EO. Hallux valgus correction with proximal metatarsal osteotomy: two-year follow-up. Foot Ankle 1992;13(6):321–6.
49. Bar-David T, Greenburg PM. Retrospective analysis of the Mau osteotomy and effect of a fibular sesamoidectomy. J Foot Ankle Surg 1998;37(3):212–6.
50. Neese DJ, Zelichowski JE, Patton GW. Mau osteotomy: an alternative procedure to the closing abductory base wedge osteotomy. J Foot Surg 1982;28(4):352–62.
51. Deorio JK, Ware AW. Single absorbable polydioxanone pin fixation for distal chevron bunion osteotomies. Foot Ankle Int 2001;22:832–5.

52. Zettl R, Trnka HJ, Easley M, et al. Moderate to severe hallux valgus deformity: correction with proximal crescentic osteotomy and distal soft-tissue release. Arch Orthop Trauma Surg 2000;120:397–402.
53. Lian GJ, Markolf K, Cracchiolo A. Strength of fixation constructs for basilar osteotomies of the first metatarsal. Foot Ankle 1992;13:509.
54. Jones C, Coughlin M, Villadot R, et al. Proximal crescentic metatarsal osteotomy: the effect of saw blade orientation on first ray elevation. Foot Ankle Int 2005;26:152–7.
55. Hyer CF, Glover JP, Berlet GC, et al. A comparison of the crescentic and Mau osteotomies for correction of hallux valgus. J Foot Ankle Surg 2008;47(2): 103–11.
56. Cohen M, Roman A, Ayres M, et al. The crescentic shelf osteotomy. J Foot Ankle Surg 1993;33:204–26.
57. Gallentine JW, DeOrio JK, DeOrio MJ. Bunion surgery using locking-plate fixation of proximal metatarsal chevron osteotomies. Foot Ankle Int 2007;28(3): 361–8.
58. Trnka HJ, Parks BG, Ivanic G, et al. Six first metatarsal shaft osteotomies: mechanical and immobilization comparisons. Clin Orthop Relat Res 2000;381: 256–65.
59. Acevedo JI, Sammarco VJ, Boucher HR, et al. Mechanical comparison of cyclic loading in five different first metatarsal shaft osteotomies. Foot Ankle Int 2002; 23(8):711–6.
60. Ludloff K. Die beseitigung des hallux valgus durch die schraege planta-dorsale osteotomie des metatarsus. Arch Klin Chir 1918;110:364–87 [in German].
61. Trnka HJ, Hofstaetter SG, Hofstaetter JG, et al. Intermediate-term results of the Ludloff osteotomy in one hundred and eleven feet. J Bone Joint Surg Am 2008; 90:531–9.
62. Resch S, Stenstrom A, Egund N. Proximal closing wedge osteotomy and adductor tenotomy for treatment of hallux valgus. Foot Ankle 1989;9:272–80.
63. Trnka HJ, Muhlbauer M, Zembsch A, et al. Basal closing wedge osteotomy for correction of hallux valgus and metatarsus primus varus: 10–22 year follow-up. Foot Ankle Int 1999;20:171–7.
64. Zembsch A, Trnka HJ, Ritschl P. Correction of hallux valgus. Metatarsal osteotomy versus excision arthroplasty. Clin Orthop 2000;376:183–94.
65. Sammarco GJ, Brainard BJ, Sammarco VJ. Bunion correction using proximal chevron osteotomy. Foot Ankle 1993;14:8–14.
66. Sammarco GJ, Conti SF. Proximal chevron metatarsal osteotomy: single incision technique. Foot Ankle 1993;14:44–7.
67. Sammarco GJ, Russo-Alexi FG. Bunion correction using proximal chevron osteotomy: a single incision technique. Foot Ankle Int 1998;19:430–7.
68. Albrecht GH. The pathology and treatment of hallux valgus. Russk Vrach 1911; 10:14–9.
69. Lapidus PW. Operative correction of the metatarsus varus primus in hallux valgus. Surg Gynecol Obstet 1934;58:183–91.
70. Truslow W. Metatarsus primus varus or hallux valgus? J Bone Joint Surg 1925;7: 75–81.
71. Sangeorzan BJ, Hansen ST Jr. Modified Lapidus procedure for hallux valgus. Foot Ankle 1989;9:262–6.
72. DeVries JG, Granata JD, Hyer CF. Fixation of first tarsometatarsal arthrodesis: a retrospective comparative cohort of two techniques. Foot Ankle Int 2011;32(2): 158–62.

73. Blitz NM. Early weightbearing of the Lapidus bunionectomy: is it feasible? Clin Podiatr Med Surg 2012;29:367–81.
74. Gruber F, Sinkov VS, Bae SY, et al. Crossed screws versus dorsomedial locking plate with compression screws for first metatarsocuneiform arthrodesis: a cadaver study. Foot Ankle Int 2008;29(9):927–30.
75. Patel S, Ford LA, Etcheverry J, et al. Modified Lapidus arthrodesis: rate of nonunion in 227 cases. J Foot Ankle Surg 2004;43(1):37–42.
76. Cottom JM. Fixation of the Lapidus arthrodesis with a plantar interfragmentary screw and medial low profile locking plate. J Foot Ankle Surg 2013;52(4):465–9.
77. Scranton PE, Coetzee CJ, Carreira D. Athrodesis of the first meatarsocuneiform joint: a comparative study of fixation methods. Foot Ankle Int 2009;30:341–5.
78. Cottom JM, Rigby RB. Biomechanical comparison of a locking plate with intra-plate compression screw versus locking plate with plantar interfragmentary screw for Lapidus arthrodesis: a cadaveric study. J Foot Ankle Surg 2013; 52(3):339–42.
79. Donnenwerth MP, Borkosky SL, Abicht BP, et al. Rate of nonunion after first metatarsal-cuneiform arthrodesis using joint curettage and two crossed compression screw fixation: a systematic review. J Foot Ankle Surg 2011; 50(6):707–9.
80. Kadous A, Abdelgawad AA, Kanlic E. Deep venous thrombosis and pulmonary embolism after surgical treatment of ankle fractures: a case report and review of literature. J Foot Ankle Surg 2012;51:457–63.
81. Basile P, Cook EA, Cook JJ. Immediate weight bearing following modified Lapidus arthrodesis. J Foot Ankle Surg 2010;49(5):459–64.
82. Sorensen MD, Berlet GC, Hyer CF. Results of Lapidus arthrodesis and locked plating with early weight bearing. Foot Ankle Spec 2009;2(5):227–33.
83. Morton DJ. Hypermobility of the first metatarsal bone: the interlinking factor be-tween metatarsalgia and longitudinal arch strains. J Bone Joint Surg 1928;10: 187–96.
84. Lapidus PW. A quarter of a century of experience with the operative correction of the metatarsus varus primus in hallux valgus. Bull Hosp Joint Dis 1956;17: 404–21.
85. Lapidus PW. The author's bunion operation from 1931–1959. Clin Orthop Relat Res 1960;16:119–35.
86. Coughlin MJ, Jones CP. Hallux valgus and first ray mobility, a prospective study. J Bone Joint Surg Am 2007;89-A(9):1887–98.
87. Klaue K, Hansen ST, Masquelet AC. Clinical, quantitative assessment of first tar-sometatarsal mobility in the sagittal plane and its relation to hallux valgus defor-mity. Foot Ankle Int 1994;15:9–13.
88. Jones CP, Coughlin MJ, Pierce-Villadot R, et al. The validity and reliability of the Klaue device. Foot Ankle Int 2005;26:951–6.
89. Glasoe WM, Allen MK, Saltzman CL. First ray dorsal mobility in relation to hallux valgus deformity and first intermetatarsal angle. Foot Ankle Int 2001; 22:98–101.
90. Grebing BR, Coughlin MJ. The effect of ankle position on the exam for first ray mobility. Foot Ankle Int 2004;25:467–75.
91. Grebing BR, Coughlin MJ. Evaluation of Morton's theory of second metatarsal hypertrophy. J Bone Joint Surg Am 2004;86:1375–86.
92. Dreeben S, Mann RA. Advanced hallux valgus deformity: long-term results uti-lizing the distal soft tissue procedure and proximal metatarsal osteotomy. Foot Ankle Int 1996;17:142–4.

93. Veri JP, Pirani SP, Claridge R. Crescentic proximal metatarsal osteotomy for moderate to severe hallux valgus: a mean 12.2 year follow-up study. Foot Ankle Int 2001;22:817–22.
94. Coughlin MJ, Jones CP, Viladot R, et al. Hallux valgus and first ray mobility: a cadaveric study. Foot Ankle Int 2004;25:537–44.
95. Kim JY, Park JS, Hwang SK, et al. Mobility changes of the first ray after hallux valgus surgery: clinical results after proximal metatarsal chevron osteotomy and distal soft tissue procedure. Foot Ankle Int 2008;29:468–72.
96. King DM, Toolan BC. Associated deformities and hypermobility in hallux valgus: an investigation with weightbearing radiographs. Foot Ankle Int 2004;25:251–5.
97. Morton DJ. The human foot; its evolution, physiology and functional disorders. New York: Columbia University Press; 1935.
98. Hansen ST Jr. Hallux valgus surgery. Morton and Lapidus were right! Clin Podiatr Med Surg 1996;13:347–54.
99. Hansen ST Jr. Functional reconstruction of the foot and ankle. Philadelphia: Lippincott Williams and Wilkins; 2000. p. 221.
100. Sarrafian SK. Functional characteristics of the foot and plantar aponeurosis under tibiotalar loading. Foot Ankle 1987;8:4–18.
101. Rush SM, Christensen JC, Johnson CH. Biomechanics of the first ray. Part II: metatarsus primus varus as a cause of hypermobility. A three-dimensional kinematic analysis in a cadaver model. J Foot Ankle Surg 2000;39:68–77.
102. Green DR, Kim P. Should the Lapidus replace the closing base wedge osteotomy? Podiatry Today 2004;56–60 Malvem: HMP Communications LLC.
103. Levin S. On your toes—tensegrity for terpsichore. Foot Biomechanics and Orthotic Therapy. Dec 1–3, Las Vegas (NV). Metatarsus Primus Varus Correction 425.

Corrective Osteotomies Used in Cavus Reconstruction

J. George DeVries, DPM[a,b,*], Jeffrey E. McAlister, DPM[c]

KEYWORDS

- Pes cavus • Osteotomy • Cavovarus • Arthrodesis • First metatarsal

KEY POINTS

- Cavus and cavovarus foot types may have various etiologies, and understanding the diagnosis will help guide the treatment algorithm.
- Cavus foot pathomechanics are complicated and require the utmost work-up.
- Reconstructive osteotomy options have been described in the forefoot, midfoot, and hindfoot and must be applied based on patient needs.
- A complete reconstruction will often include osteotomies as well as tendon work and limited arthrodesis, and must be specifically tailored to each unique patient.

INTRODUCTION

Cavus foot and ankle reconstruction is complicated and must take into account many aspects of the disease and reconstruction. The etiology, flexibility, and progression need to be clinically assessed, and a full imaging and diagnostic work-up must be undertaken. Reconstructive options include soft tissue releases, lengthenings, and transfers, and most often these are accompanied with osseous correction. Depending on the needs of the patient and the pathologic features, osteotomies and arthrodeses will need to be considered. This article reviews reconstructive options, focused on the various osteotomies that can be utilized. Various options have been described in the forefoot, midfoot, and hindfoot, and often a combination or arthodesis adjunct will be performed as well.

J.G. DeVries consults with Arthrex, Inc (Naples, Florida) and receives compensation as educational faculty. J.E. McAlister has no financial or commercial conflicts of interest as it pertains to this topic. There are no sources of funding for this article.
[a] Orthopedics & Sports Medicine, BayCare Clinic, 501 North 10th Street, Manitowoc, WI 54220, USA; [b] Orthopedics & Sports Medicine, BayCare Clinic, 2020 Riverside Drive, 2nd Floor, Green Bay, WI 54301, USA; [c] Orthopedic Surgery, CORE Institute, 1615 West Red Fox Road, Phoenix, AZ 85085, USA
* Corresponding author. Orthopedics & Sports Medicine, BayCare Clinic, 501 North 10th Street, Manitowoc, WI 54220.
E-mail address: jdevries@baycare.net

ETIOLOGY

Pes cavus or cavovarus foot types may typically present in a foot and ankle surgeon's office with or without a previous diagnosis of a neuromuscular condition or similar etiology. Therefore, it is paramount to determine the underlying etiology to understand the pathology and most predictable treatment. The typical etiology for a pes cavus foot type is one of neurologic, traumatic, or idiopathic origin. Common neuromuscular disorders associated include Charcot-Marie-Tooth disease (CMT), cerebral palsy, muscular dystrophy, and other peripheral sensory motor disorders.[1,2] Traumatic cases are more easily identifiable but may result from a multitude of injury patterns in adults and children.[3]

Understanding the etiology helps determine which surgical procedures to choose based on the disease. For instance, CMT is the most common hereditary motor sensory neuropathy and causes peroneal muscle atrophy and imbalance. There are 17 types of CMT, and the most common subtype is CMT1A, which is caused by a mutation or duplication in the peripheral myelin protein-22 (PMP22) gene. Progressive weakness of the peroneus brevis and tibialis anterior myotendinous units causes a cavovarus foot type noted by an overpowering tibialis posterior and peroneus longus, respectively. The recruitment of extensor hallucis longus as tibialis anterior weakens also creates a marked increase in arch height. The symptoms of foot drop and claw-toes also will develop as the disease worsens, and a high steppage gait is noted.[4,5]

When cerebral palsy is the key diagnosis, the physician must be aware of the spastic deformities, which occur as the most common form of the nonprogressive condition. Pes cavus and cavovarus foot deformities are usually accompanied by ankle equinus as well. Muscular imbalances are a critical component and involve the gastrocnemius–soleal complex, tibialis posterior, and tibialis anterior. Beyond the scope of this article, but prudent to understand, are the orthopedic deformities present in a patient diagnosed with cerebral palsy. The key is getting the diagnosis early in childhood and treating these patients with soft-tissue releases and tendon transfers. If the disease is in its later stages and becomes more rigid, oftentimes large osseous procedures and arthrodeses are performed.

Many forms of trauma can result in a cavovarus attitude of the foot and or ankle depending on the severity and level of incident. A subtle history of repetitive ankle sprains can result in significant injury to the peroneus brevis, which would in turn, allow compensation of the peroneus longus and increase in a forefoot deformity. Compartment syndrome in the deep compartment of the lower leg can result in a contracture of the tibialis posterior and flexor digitorum longus and flexor hallucis longus causing an irreducible cavovarus deformity at multiple levels. One complication related to talar neck fractures is a varus malunion, which locks the midtarsal joint and supinates the hindfoot significantly, causing forefoot compensation with a plantarflexed first ray.[3]

CAVUS BIOMECHANICS

Understanding the biomechanical component of each individual deformity is paramount and often difficult in a cavus foot or an ankle varus with a compensatory hindfoot. Biomechanically, a cavus foot type can be categorized into several different categories, and this helps the surgeon delineate the procedure of choice.

The common breakdown of cavus foot types is anterior, posterior, and mixed. Anterior cavus foot types may be flexible or rigid, and the apex of the deformity is seen at the tarsometatarsal or lesser tarsal joints. An associated pathology is metatarsus adductus, whereby all 5 metatarsals are in a valgus orientation and may present with a skew or Z-type forefoot. The first ray is also seen at a greater inclination to the lesser metatarsals in some patients with anterior cavus. Posterior cavus is seen with an increased calcaneal pitch of greater than 30° from the weightbearing surface. This also causes the calcaneus to invert in the frontal plane, because the pull of the Achilles tendon is medial, and the first ray and forefoot compensate into supination. These deformities exist most often in parallel, and the cavus component may either be forefoot-driven or hindfoot-driven as a result.[6]

PHYSICAL EXAMINATION

Patients with a cavus or cavovarus foot deformity will present with various pathologies, but most commonly lateral ankle and/or foot pain. It is imperative to examine these deformities in full with a patient in a seated and standing position and also assess their gait pattern. Each cycle of the gait is important in the overall deformity. Swing phase may exhibit a foot drop, worsening claw toes, or an uncompensated hindfoot varus. Stance phase may reveal claw toes, hindfoot varus, or a plantarflexed first ray. Presence of hypertrophic lesions or calluses is typically a sign of increased load and can assist in diagnosis. It may also be helpful to examine shoe wear patterns to better ascertain the increased load during gait (**Fig. 1**).[7]

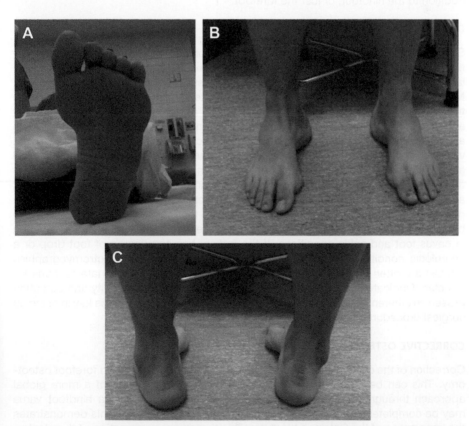

Fig. 1. (A–C) Clinical pictures of a typical cavovarus foot. (A) Plantar view demonstrates callus formation specifically at the heel, first and fifth metatarsal heads. (B) Anterior view demonstrates accentuation of the medial arch and peek-a-boo heel. (C) Hindfoot alignment view shows calcaneal varus and fat pad hypertrophy of the first metatarsal head.

Certain deformities are exacerbated with a tendon contracture. Equinus may play a particularly important role in a patient's deformity and should be noted during the physical examination. The basic Silfverskiold test will assist the clinician in determining the level of equinus with the knee bent and extended. Psuedoequinus may also be present and is the result of a decrease in talar declination leading to early impingement of the talus on the distal tibia in dorsiflexion. Peroneal tendinopathy should also be assessed with manual muscle testing of both peroneus longus and brevis. Typically, chronic tears or rupture of the peroneus brevis may result in an overpowered peroneus longus tendon and first ray plantarflexion. This may lead to a forefoot valgus and increased hindfoot varus. In addition to muscle testing of all tendons, a complete neurologic examination is paramount and has unique importance in cavovarus deformities.

The Coleman block test is a key diagnostic tool utilized in cavovarus foot types.[8] The lateral forefoot is placed on a wooden block, which allows the medial forefoot to be unloaded, and the foot is visualized from posterior. The practitioner is looking for a correction of hindfoot varus as the lateral forefoot is placed on the block. If the hindfoot varus does not correct out of varus and into a more neutral position, then the forefoot is not the only contributing factor to the deformity, but the hindfoot is in a fixed position. This will help determine whether a forefoot deformity needs to be corrected in addition to the hindfoot, or just the forefoot.

DIAGNOSTICS

Standard weight-bearing foot and ankle radiographs are utilized during the examination along with a long-leg axial view or calcaneal axial view. Various angles are calculated for determining the severity of the deformity such as, calcaneal inclination angle, Meary angle, and Hobb angle.[9] On an anteroposterior foot view, one can appreciate the degree of transverse plane deformity such as forefoot adduction or midfoot adduction. The calcaneal axial view is a important view to look for calcaneal varus and assist in preoperative planning for a lateral calcaneal wedge. On a lateral foot view, one is able to assess for the degree of plantarflexion of the first ray or metatarsal and determine the amount of correction needed in the forefoot. Advanced imaging is used to view periarticular pathology, but also grade articular damage in the midfoot and hindfoot. Computed tomography (CT) is typically ordered when determining the degree of arthritis and subchondral cysts within the involved joints. MRI may also be utilized if one is concerned for ligamentous or tendon pathology, which is common in cavus foot and ankle conditions. If the patient has any degree of foot drop or a neurologic condition, nerve conduction velocities (NCVs) and electromyographies (EMGs) are often helpful in determining the diagnosis and appropriate tendons for transfer, if indicated. The cavus foot and ankle is a complex deformity and can often present in different ways, so utilizing the appropriate diagnostic tools is key in planning surgical procedures and overall treatment.

CORRECTIVE OSTEOTOMIES OF THE CAVUS FOREFOOT

Correction of the cavus deformity may need to be addressed through forefoot osteotomy. This can be as a primary corrective procedure, or as part of a more global approach through the hindfoot. Occasionally patients who have a hindfoot varus may be completely reducible when removing the forefoot forces. This demonstrates the importance of the Coleman block test.[8] In these cases, correction of the plantarflexed first ray may correct the hindfoot deformity and no longer necessitate further bony work in the hindfoot. Conversely, a pronounced hindfoot or ankle varus deformity will overload the lateral forefoot and early on will offload the medial column. As the condition persists, there may be a compensatory plantarflexion of the medial forefoot in order to balance the forefoot. In these cases, after the hindfoot deformity is corrected, the patient can be left with a significant residual forefoot valgus, that, if rigid, will need be addressed in order to align the forefoot to the hindfoot.

Care must be taken to assess the forefoot to determine the specific location of deformity. An anterior cavus deformity can consist of plantarflexion of all the metatarsals at the tarsal–metatarsal level.[10–12] Correction may need to address multiple metatarsals. More commonly the deformity is most pronounced at the 1st metatarsal. This common issue is often caused by CMT, when the peroneus longus is functional, but the tibialis anterior is not. This results in an unopposed peroneus longus and plantarflextion of the first ray. This will lead to a forefoot valgus, and can drive a hindfoot varus. When this is the specific location of deformity, an isolated dorsiflexory first metatarsal osteotomy may be more indicated.

Osteotomy of the metatarsals is rarely done in isolation. Obtaining adequate excursion of the metatarsals in a dorsiflexory position will at least require a release of the plantar fascia or complete Steindler stripping. This will release the tension band effect of the plantar foot soft tissue structures, which can bind the metatarsals in a plantarflexed position. The peroneus longus may need to be released, lengthened, or transferred to remove the deforming pull. In addition, even if the forefoot is the driving force causing a hindfoot varus, the hindfoot deformity may need to be addressed. This can be in the form of tendon transfers in supple deformity, or in the case of a rigid deformity, osteotomies or arthrodeses may be required. The forefoot osteotomy is most often 1 aspect of a more complete cavus reconstruction.

In cases that entail primarily a plantarflexion of the first metatarsal, either in isolation or in the face of hindfoot pathology, an isolated dorsiflexory first metatarsal osteotomy may be performed. This is a common procedure performed, particularly in the face of a Coleman block test that reveals a forefoot-driven hindfoot varus. By elevating the first metatarsal in isolation, this will correct the plantarflexion of the medial column, but also will de-rotate a forefoot valgus. This de-rotation will correct the common coronal plane deformity seen in cavus feet, particularly in CMT.[13]

The dorsiflexory first ray wedge osteotomy is performed with an incision starting over the medial cunieform and extending along the long axis of the first metatarsal. The incicion is parallel with extensor tendon. Dissection is carried deep to the extensor hallucis longus tendon, and the sheath is opened and the tendon is mobilized medially or laterally. The periosteum over the base of the first metatarsal is opened, and the osteotomy is made. The proximal cut is made approximately 1 cm distal and parallel to the first tarsometatarsal joint. The second osteotomy cut is made distal and converging on the plantar cortex. Care is taken to ensure that the plantar cortex remains intact, and the osteotomy is hinged, or greensticked plantarly. Plantar pressure along the first metatarsal head is applied, and the ankle is dorsiflexed into a rectus position. The forefoot position is assessed according to the long axis of the tibia, and must be perpendicular to this, provided there is no tibial deformity. If there is residual forefoot valgus, further resection of the dorsally based wedge is undertaken. Once adequate correction has taken place, the osteotomy is fixated. This can be performed with an oblique screw through the osteotomy, but is more often fixated with dorsal fixation. This can be a dorsal plate, staple, or tension band (**Fig. 2**).[14,15]

When forefoot deformity is truly seen throughout the forefoot at the tarsal–metatarsal level, multiple metatarsal osteotomies may be required. This is the case in a true sagittal plane deformity, with less coronal plane malalignment than is seen with the plantarflexed first ray. Incisions are made to access the metatarsals to be included for osteotomy. A longitudanal incision is made between the second and third

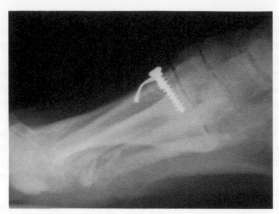

Fig. 2. Dorsiflexory 1st metatarsal osteotomy fixated with tension banded cerclage wire. This method depends on the plantar hinge remaining intact and tension side mechanics. It may be inadequate in the event of plantar cortex violation.

metatarsals, and between the fourth and fifth metatarsals to access these specific metatarsals. The osteotomy and fixation are carried out as described previously.[10–12,16]

In addition to closing wedge osteotomies of the metatarsals, plantar opening wedge osteotomy of the cuneiforms has been described as well, and this can be done in conjunction with closing wedges of the metatarsals. This has been primarily been reported in a pediatric population, and has not been widely adopted for use in an adult population. The incisional approach is directly medial, and then a distractor is used to open the osteotomy. Graft material is inserted, and this can be donated from the closing wedge from the metatarsals. Fixation is achieved with Kirschner wire fixation or can be with a medial plate.[17–19]

CORRECTIVE OSTEOTOMY OF THE CAVUS MIDFOOT

Understanding the apex of the deformity is paramount in the midfoot correction, which is visualized on a weight bearing lateral foot view. The deformity is typically not only in the midfoot, forefoot, or hindfoot, but a combination of the three. Therefore, an isolated osseous procedure in the midfoot will not correct a forefoot valgus or a fixed hindfoot varus. The midfoot deformities are typically performed with procedures such as a Cole, Jahss, or Japas osteotomy.[20] These are performed at the apex of the deformity in the midfoot. As described in previous paragraphs, to reduce the deformity in an appropriate order of progression is also important. Typically, a midfoot osteotomy would be performed after a hindfoot correction or hindfoot osteotomy and plantar fascia release but before a forefoot procedure.

Several osteotomies exist and have been described in previous reports, but the common procedures are described here. A Cole osteotomy, as described by Saunders and Cole[21] is a dorsal midfoot wedge resection, which reduces anterior cavus and global cavus. The osteotomy is performed through a single midfoot, midline approach retracting the deep neurovascular structures. Authors have described a dual incision approach to allow for a large skin island or bridge and accommodate the osteotomy as well. The osteotomy begins medially at the naviculo-cuneiform joint and ends within the lateral cuboid. A large sagittal saw is then used to take a 1–1.5 cm dorsal wedge from the midfoot. Specific care is taken to avoid the talonavicular and calcaneocuboid joints. The amount of wedge removed can be predetermined on a lateral foot view but is typically determined intraoperatively. Reduction of the deformity is performed with dorsiflexion of the forefoot and metatarsals on the hindfoot. The key to this procedure is performing a Steindler stripping or plantar fascia release prior to correction to allow for easier manipulation. While manually maintaining reduction, the osteotomy is fixated with multiple points of temporary fixation. Final fixation if obtained after confirmation under fluoroscopy is performed. This may be done with screws, plates, or staples, as the surgeon desires. Locked compression plates are great options, as well as 4.0 mm partially threaded cortical screws. Patients are kept nonweight-bearing for 8 to 10 weeks or until radiographic signs of healing are seen. Complications are not uncommon. Nonunion, malunion, hardware failure, and wound dehiscence have all been reported.[1,10] This osteotomy is not to be taken lightly, and the architecture of the foot is significantly altered and shortened. Few reports have been published on the functional outcomes of this type of midfoot osteotomy for cavus foot reconstruction. Mendicino and colleagues reported on 11 feet in 8 patients after a midfoot dorsiflexion osteotomy with a mean follow-up of 23 months. A change of 16° was seen on a lateral foot radiograph of the talo-first metatarsal angle and no reported complications. Eighty percent of the patients said they would recommend this procedure to others (**Fig. 3**).[22]

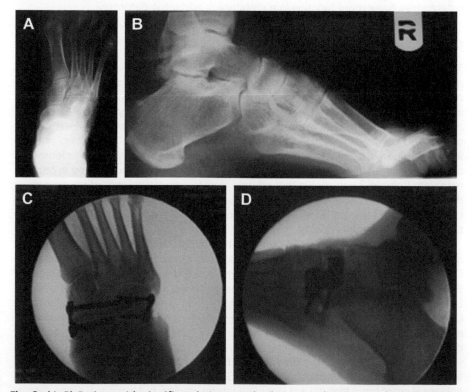

Fig. 3. (*A–D*) Patient with significantly increased calcaneal inclination angle and midfoot deformity with concomitant clawtoes. (*A, B*) are preoperative radiographic views of a cavovarus foot type. Planned procedures included plantar fascia release, posterior soft tissue release, midfoot wedge resection, Jones tenosuspension with clawtoe corrections. (*C, D*) Dual incision midfoot approach was utilized for plate fixation. (*Courtesy of* D. Blacklidge, DPM, Carmel, IN.)

To prevent the inherent shortening of the foot with a dorsiflexion midfoot osteotomy, a V-shaped osteotomy may also be performed at the apex of the deformity, as originally described by Japas.[23] This osteotomy was described with the apex proximal, at the lateral navicular bone, and ending laterally in the cuboid and medially in the medial cuneiform. A similar plantar soft tissue release is also prudent prior to reduction of this osteotomy. No bone excision is performed during the reduction as the forefoot is elevated on the hindfoot and fixated appropriately. This procedure is technically challenging and not typically advocated over a Cole osteotomy. The same type of complications can occur with this osteotomy including malunion, nonunion, and residual pain. Chatterjee and Sahu reported on 18 adolescents with paralytic cavus deformities. With a 5-year follow-up, only 4 patients required further procedures, such as calcaneal osteotomies.[24]

Jahss has described a tarsometatarsal truncated wedge arthrodesis, which is uncommonly performed as a single entity for anterior cavus.[20] The difficulty with this arthrodesis is the potential for imbalance of the metatarsal heads, nonunions, and the hardware removal. Again, this arthrodesis procedure is more of historical note and not a standard practice in most clinics.

Various authors have described isolated cuboid and cuneiform osteotomies, albeit their indications are limited and have not been shown to be significantly useful.[25] Isolated lateral column shortening osteotomies help to reduce the hindfoot varus. These osteotomies have more function in a metatarsus adductus deformity.

CORRECTIVE OSTEOTOMY OF THE CAVUS HINDFOOT

The hindfoot may demonstrate irreducible varus deformity in some cases. Patients will maintain a varus alignment of the hindfoot during the Coleman block test. This can be caused by a true deformity or contracture that originates in the hindfoot. Conversely, if a forefoot-driven cavus is left untreated long enough, a previously reducible deformity may become rigid and require a calcaneal osteotomy. The goals of a calcaneal osteotomy are to convert the Achilles to an everting force, lateralize the ground reactive forces, and can also be used to reduce the calcaneal inclination. These osteotomies are capable of reducing forces in the ankle, and have been demonstrated in cadaver research. Schmid[26] has shown that a 5 mm and 10 mm lateral shift of the calcaneus resulted in a 2 mm and 3 mm shift in force distribution and 41% and 49% reduction in peak pressure at the ankle, respectively. A much smaller effect on pressure distribution is seen in the subtalar joint.[27]

The most widely used osteotomy used for hindfoot correction of varus malalignment is the lateral closing wedge calcaneal osteotomy. Originally this was described by Dwyer and was isolated as a closing wedge that left the medial cortex in place.[28] By closing the osteotomy down laterally, the calcaneal tuberosity is shifted laterally. Later modifications of this osteotomy include a through and through osteotomy. Once completed, the posterior tuber can be shifted as well. This can be shifted proximally to reduce the calcaneal inclination. This type of correction was originally described as a crescentic osteotomy by Samilson,[29] but can now easily be performed with a linear osteotomy and rigidly internally fixated. Similarly, the tuber can be shifted laterally to increase the reduction of varus. Suppan[30] described a modification of this calcaneal osteotomy that did not include a lateral wedge, but a coronal plane derotation combined with a shift both superiorly and laterally. This basic osteotomy through the posterior tuber of the calcaneus has been found to be very useful, and modifications allow correction of almost any specific deformity that needs to be addressed during reconstruction (**Fig. 4**).

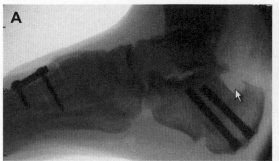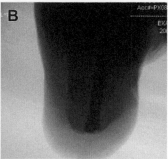

Fig. 4. (A, B) Modification of Dwyer calcaneal osteotomy with through and through cut with lateral and proximal slide. This was used in combination with dorsiflexory first metatarsal osteotomy, plantar fascial release, and side-to-side peroneal tendon anastomosis. Plate fixation of the first metatarsal was utilized because of plantar cortex violation.

The procedure is approached through a lateral approach to the calcaneus. An oblique incision measuring approximately 7 cm is made in a linear fashion posterior and inferior to the peroneal tendons. Care is taken to avoid the sural nerve or calcaneal branch of the sural nerve. Once this is identified, dissection is carried deep to the lateral calcaneal wall, and the periosteum is incised along the line of the osteotomy. More dissection than is needed for a medial displacement calcaneal osteotomy is necessary in order to facilitate the removal of a wedge of bone. The first osteotomy is made from superior–posterior proceeding inferior–anterior. The saw is brought up to the medial cortex, but care is taken to avoid penetrating this cortex. The second osteotomy is made parallel to the first osteotomy, converging medially at the medial calcaneal wall. The wedge of bone is removed from the incision, and the osteotomy is closed down. If no shift is needed of the calcaneal tuber, the osteotomy can be fixated with staples, plates, or axial screws delivered percutaneously for the posterior aspect of the heel. Guidewires in the posterior tuber can be used as a lever to toggle the osteotomy closed if it does not easily do so. Variations of the wedge, direction, and orientation of the Dwyer osteotomy have been examined for effect of varus correction, shortening, and shift of the pull of the Achilles.[31–33] Results have been generally positive for lateral calcaneal slides or wedges in the literature.[13]

In order to provide a shift of the posterior tuber, the osteotomy is completed through the medial cortex, usually after the wedge has been removed. The surfaces are reciprocally planed to ensure excellent apposition of the osteotomy after the shift. A purely dorsal shift can be fixated in any of the ways described. A lateral shift will require axial screw fixation or specialized plates or staples that have a step-off incorporated in them. This can be used as a template to ensure adequate shift, and some plates can actually facilitate the shift (Fig. 5).

A calcaneal scarf osteotomy has been described as well, and has been shown to be a versatile corrective option in the hindfoot.[34–36] Originally described by Malerba, it has been described as a correction or varus or valgus calcaneal deformity. Exposure is undertaken through a lateral curvilinear incision inferior to the peroneal tendons. Exposure is carried deep through the subcutaneous tissues, again with care to avoid the sural nerve as well as the peroneal tendons. Once dissection is carried to the calcaneus, the lateral wall is exposed, and the osteotomy is planned. In general, the osteotomy entails 3 bone cuts. There is a posterior–superior cut that exits on the dorsal aspect of the posterior tuber, posterior to the subtalar joint, a central osteotomy

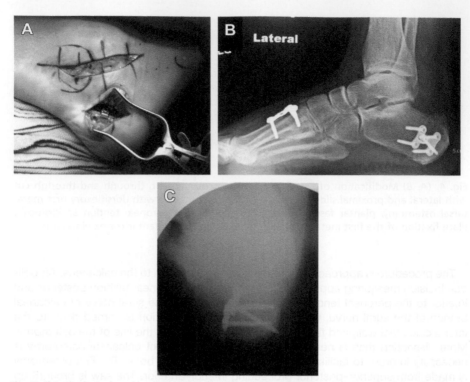

Fig. 5. (A–C) Clinical and radiographic image of plate fixation allowing for lateral translation of Dwyer calcaneal osteotomy. This was done in conjunction with Brostrum lateral ankle stabilization, plantar fascial release, and dorsiflexory first metatarsal osteotomy.

that runs along the longitudinal axis of the body of the calcaneus, and a distal osteotomy that exits plantarly, proximal to the calcaneal cuboid joint. Various angles of the intersections of the osteotomies have been suggested, and wedges can be inserted or removed to help aid correction. In the case of a cavus correction, the posterior tuber can be slid laterally; a lateral wedge can be removed from the central osteotomy to correct varus, or a rectangular section of bone can be removed from this area to slide the posterior tuber proximally to improve calcaneal inclination.[34,37]

CORRECTIVE ARTHRODESIS IN THE CAVUS FOOT

This article focused on osteotomies for correction of the cavus foot. These corrective bony cuts can be used in the face of a supple deformity without arthritis in the joint. However, if the deformity is severe, progressive, or rigid, arthrodesis through the joint may be necessary. This has been described through every segment of the foot. Medial column arthrodesis[38] and fusion through all the tarsometatarsal joints[20] has been described. A hindfoot double arthrodesis through the talonavicular and calcaneal–cuboid joints[39] can correct specific deformity at this level, and a triple arthrodesis[40,41] is a powerful, predictable, and classical procedure for multiplanar cavus foot correction in the hindfoot. As the deformity and arthritis progress, ankle, tibiotalocalcaneal, or even pantalar arthrodesis may become needed. Often a complete cavus correction will entail osteotomies and arthrodeses in combination as the deformity necessitates.

AUTHORS' PREFERRED TECHNIQUE

No cavus foot is the same, and therefore no 1 surgical approach can be uniformly applied in the reconstructive approach. The Coleman block test is one of the most important tools that physicians have when approaching the cavus foot, but certainly it cannot be the only tool used. Ankle films must uniformly be taken to assess any arthritis, instability, or incongruity at the tibiotalar joint. Hindfoot alignment films are useful to measure the deformity and directly see the relationship of the hindfoot and tibia.[42] Advanced imaging must be considered to assess the condition of the joints involved, as well as the tendons about the ankle. Additional studies may include EMGs or ultrasound evaluation.

Beyond fully imaging the cavus foot, assessment of progression and instability is crucial. Care must be taken to identify areas that may lead to recurrence, and these must be addressed accordingly. Even a well-performed reconstructive procedure may eventually become symptomatic if the underlying deforming forces are not addressed. Balancing of soft tissue structures is paramount to success, and this may mean releases, lengthenings, or transfers. These procedures have been explored at length in the literature and will need to be part of any successful procedure in the long-term follow-up. Although this article focused on osteotomies for the correction of the cavus foot, judicious use of joint arthrodesis needs to be part of the surgical algorithm. This can be due to the presence of arthritis in the joint, rigidity of the deformity, magnitude of the deformity, or concern for progression.

Understanding that no single answer to cavus reconstruction can be given, the authors have common approaches to the various levels of approach, but these need to be comprehensive and tailored to the specific patient needs. A truly isolated forefoot cavus with a plantarflexed first ray and valgus forefoot can often be addressed with a dorsiflexory osteotomy of the first metatarsal to eliminate the valgus forefoot, a plantar fascial release or Steindler stripping to release any tether to the plantar foot and first metatarsal, and release of the peroneus longus at the cuboid tunnel with side-to-side anastomosis with the peroneus brevis to remove the plantarflexory deforming force. Dorsiflexory fusion of the first tarsometarsal joint can be undertaken as the magnitude of deformity increases or in the presence of arthritis. As the deformity persists and progresses, the hindfoot will need to be addressed. Early in the progression, a true Dwyer lateral calcaneal wedge osteotomy may need to be added to the previously mentioned procedures to correct the hindfoot alignment. If a simple wedge is unable to correct the deformity, the osteotomy is completed and shifted laterally along with the wedge removal. For more hindfoot-related deformity without ankle involvement, a triple arthrodesis may be necessary in the reconstruction. Forefoot alignment with metatarsal osteotomy is undertaken to rebalance the forefoot to the hindfoot. Most often a posterior tibial tendon transfer is added to the cuboid or lateral cuneiformy to remove its deforming force.

Cavus foot reconstruction is complicated and requires a dynamic approach. Osteotomies to help complete the correction have been described and are used throughout the forefoot, midfoot, and hindfoot. Appropriate use of these osteotomies, in conjunction to soft tissue rebalancing and judicious use of arthrodeses, can lead to successful cavus foot corrective surgery.

REFERENCES

1. Alexander IJ, Johnson KA. Assessment and management of pes cavus in Charcot-Marie-Tooth disease. Clin Orthop 1989;246:273–81.

2. Tenuta J, Shelton YA, Miller F. Long term follow-up of triple arthrodesis in patients with cerebral palsy. J Pediatr Orthop 1993;13:713–6.

3. Sangeorzan BJ, Wagner UA, Harrington RM, et al. Contact characteristics of the subtalar joint: the effect of talar neck misalignment. J Orthop Res 1992;10: 544–51.

4. Mann RA, Missirian J. Pathophysiology of Charcot-Marie-Tooth disease. Clin Orthop Relat Res 1988;234:221–8.

5. Tynan MC, Klenerman L, Helliwell TR, et al. Investigation of muscle imbalance in the leg in symptomatic forefoot pes cavus: a mulitdiscipinary study. Foot Ankle 1992;13:489–500.

6. Smith TF, Green DR. Pes cavus. In: Banks AS, Downey MS, Martin DE, et al, editors. McGlamry's comprehensive textbook of foot and ankle surgery. 3rd edition. Philadelphia: Lippincott Williams & Wilkins; 2001. p. 765–7.

7. Deben SE, Pomeroy GC. Subtle cavus foot: diagnosis and management. J Am Acad Orthop Surg 2014;22(8):512–20.

8. Coleman SS, Chesnut WJ. A simple test for hindfoot flexibility in the cavovarus foot. Clin Orthop Relat Res 1977;123:60–2.

9. Perera A, Guha A. Clinical and radiographic evaluation of the cavus foot: surgical implications. Foot Ankle Clin 2013;18(4):619–28.

10. Watanabe RS. Metatarsal osteotomy for the cavus foot. Clin Orthop 1990;252: 217–30.

11. Gould N. Surgery in advanced Charcot-Marie-Tooth disease. Foot Ankle 1984;4: 267–73.

12. Bacardi BE, Alm WA. Modifications of the Gould operation for cavo-varus reconstruction of the foot. J Foot Surg 1988;25:181–7.

13. Guyton GP, Mann RA. Pes cavus. In: Coughlin MJ, Mann RA, Saltzmann CL, editors. Surgery of the foot and ankle. 8th edition. Philadelphia: Mosby Elsevier; 2007. p. 1139–41.

14. Leeuwesteijn AE, de Visser E, Louwerens JW. Flexible cavo varus feet in Charcot-Marie-Tooth disease treated with first ray osteotomy combined with soft tissue surgery: a short-term to mid-term outcome study. Foot Ankle Surg 2010;16: 142–7.

15. Sammarco GJ, Taylor R. Combined calcaneal and metatarsal osteotomies for the treatment of cavus foot. Foot Ankle Clin 2001;6(3):533–43.

16. Wang GJ, Shaffer LW. Osteotomy of the metatarsals for pes cavus. South J Med 1977;70:77–9.

17. Mubarak SJ, Van Valin SE. Osteotomies of the foot for cavus deformities in children. J Pediatr Orthop 2009;29(3):294–9.

18. Fowler SB, Brooks AL, Parrish TF. The cavo-varus foot. J Bone Joint Surg Am 1959;41A:757.

19. Wicart P, Seringe R. Plantar opening wedge osteotomy of cuneiform bones combined with selective plantar release and Dwyer osteotomy for pes cavovarus in children. J Pediatr Orthop 2006;26(1):100–8.

20. Jahss MH. Tarsometatarsal truncated-wedge arthrodesis for pes cavus and equinovarus deformity of the fore part of the foot. J Bone Joint Surg Am 1980;62: 713–22.

21. Cole WH. The classic. The treatment of claw-foot. By Wallace H. Cole. 1940. Clin Orthop Relat Res 1983;181:3–6.

22. Tullis BL, Mendicino RW, Catanzariti AR, et al. The Cole midfoot osteotomy: a retrospective review of 11 procedures in 8 patients. J Foot Ankle Surg 2004; 43(3):160–5.

23. Japas LM. Surgical treatment of pes cavus by tarsal V-osteotomy. Preliminary report. J Bone Joint Surg Am 1968;50(5):927–44.
24. Chatterjee P, Sahu MK. A prospective study of Japas' osteotomy in paralytic pes cavus deformity in adolescent feet. Indian J Orthop 2009;43(3):281–5.
25. Ingram AJ. Paralytic disorders. In: Crenshaw AH, editor. Campbell's orthopaedics, vol. 4, 7th edition. St Louis (MO): Mosby; 1987. p. 2925–3061.
26. Schmid T, Zurbriggen S, Zderic I, et al. Ankle joint pressure changes in pes cavovarus model: supramalleolar valgus osteotomy versus lateralizing calcaneal osteotomy. Foot Ankle Int 2013;34(9):1190–7.
27. Krause FG, Sutter D, Waehnert D, et al. Ankle joint pressure changes in a pes cavovarus model after lateralizing calcaneal osteotomies. Foot Ankle Int 2010; 31(9):741–6.
28. Dwyer FC. Osteotomy of the calcaneum for pes cavus. J Bone Joint Surg Br 1959;41:80–6.
29. Samilson RL. Crescentic osteotomy of the os calsis for calcaneocavus feet. In: Bateman JE, editor. Foot science. Philadelphia: WB Saunders; 1976. p. 18.
30. Suppan RJ. Surgery for congenital deformities of the feet. Clin Podiatry 1984;1: 667–707.
31. Kraus JC, Fischer MT, McCormick JJ, et al. Geometry of the lateral sliding, closing wedge calcaneal osteotomy: review of the two methods and technical tip to minimize shortening. Foot Ankle Int 2014;35(3):238–42.
32. Krackow KA, Hales D, Jones L. Preoperative planning and surgical technique for performing a Dwyer calcaneal osteotomy. J Pediatr Orthop 1985;5(2):214–8.
33. Lamm BM, Gesheff MG, Salton HL, et al. Preoperative planning and intraoperative technique for accurate realignment of the Dwyer calcaneal osteotomy. J Foot Ankle Surg 2012;51(6):743–8.
34. Malerba F, De MArchi F. Calcaneal osteotomies. Foot Ankle Clin 2005;10(3): 523–40.
35. Feuerstein CA, Weil L Jr, Weil LS Sr, et al. The calcaneal scark osteotomy: surgical correction of the adult acquired flatfoot deformity and radiographic results. Foot Ankle Spec 2013;6(5):367–71.
36. Knupp M, Pagenstert G, Valderrabano V, et al. Osteotomies in varus malalignment of the ankle. Oper Orthop Traumatol 2008;20(3):262–73.
37. Weil LS Jr, Roukis TS. The calcaneal scarf osteotomy: operative technique. J Foot Ankle Surg 2001;40(3):178–82.
38. McElvenny RT, Caldwell GD. A new operation for correction of cavus foot: fusion of first metatarsocuneiform navicular joints. Clin Orthop 1958;11:85–92.
39. Clain MR, Baxter DE. Simultaneous calcaneocuboid and talonavicular fusion. J Bone Joint Surg Br 1994;76B:133–6.
40. Ryerson EW. Arthrodesing operations on the feet. J Bone Joint Surg Am 1923;5: 453–79.
41. Siffert RS, del Torto U. "Beak" triple arthrodesis for sever cavus deformity. Clin Orthop Relat Res 1983;181:65–7.
42. Saltzman CL, El-Khoury GY. The hindfoot alignment view. Foot Ankle Int 1995; 16(9):572–6.

Osteotomies for the Flexible Adult Acquired Flatfoot Disorder

Kyle S. Peterson, DPM, AACFAS[a],*,
Benjamin D. Overley Jr, DPM, FACFAS[b], Thomas C. Beideman, DPM[c]

KEYWORDS

- Posterior tibial tendon dysfunction • Adult acquired flatfoot disorder
- Calcaneal osteotomy • Koutsogiannis • Evans • Malerba • Cotton

KEY POINTS

- Stage II adult acquired flatfoot disorder is often surgically treated with joint-sparing osteotomies of the calcaneus and medial column.
- Traditional osteotomies of the calcaneus involve a medial displacement of the posterior tuberosity or a lengthening of the anterior calcaneus.
- Newer techniques now incorporate both a medial calcaneal slide and lateral column lengthening through 1 Z osteotomy of the calcaneus (Malerba osteotomy).
- If forefoot supinatus exists with the flexible flatfoot, a medial cuneiform opening wedge osteotomy (Cotton osteotomy) can be performed.

 Video fixation of the posterior calcaneal arm accompanies this article at www. podiatric.theclinics.com/

INTRODUCTION

Adult acquired flatfoot disorder (AAFD) is a debilitating musculoskeletal condition frequently seen by foot and ankle specialists. Posterior tibial tendon dysfunction (PTTD) is the primary cause for the development of a flatfoot deformity in an adult.[1] Reconstruction of the flatfoot deformity with joint-sparing osteotomies is typically performed in Johnson and Strom stage II PTTD.[2] Stage II PTTD is depicted by a flexible flatfoot deformity with hindfoot valgus, forefoot abduction, and forefoot varus. The goal of reconstructive surgery is to create a pain-free, well-aligned plantigrade foot

The authors have nothing to disclose for this article.
[a] Suburban Orthopaedics, 1110 West Schick Road, Bartlett, IL 60103, USA; [b] Division of Orthopedics, Pottstown Medical Specialists, Inc, 1610 Medical Drive, Pottstown, PA 19464, USA; [c] Mercy Suburban Hospital, 2701 Dekalb Pike, Norristown, PA 19401, USA
* Corresponding author.
E-mail address: kyle.s.pete@gmail.com

that removes tension from the posterior tibial tendon and lessens the progression of hindfoot arthritis and deformity. This article discusses the preoperative planning, operative approach, surgical technique, fixation options, and postoperative course for osteotomies used in the treatment of flexible flatfoot deformities.

HISTORICAL PERSPECTIVE

Calcaneal osteotomies have been described for the treatment of flexible hindfoot valgus deformities. Gleich described the first calcaneal osteotomy in 1893, in which a plantar-medial closing base wedge was performed to increase the calcaneal inclination angle.[3] The medial displacement calcaneal osteotomy (MDCO) became popular in 1971 as introduced by Koutsogiannis (**Fig. 1**).[4] In 1975, Evans described a lateral column lengthening procedure offering triplane correction in pes planovalgus (**Fig. 2**).[5] Many modifications have been made to these osteotomies through the years with varying recommendations for fixation, surgical approach, and technique.

Long-term studies after Evans procedures indicate that calcaneocuboid joint (CCJ) arthritis is a common complication. To combat this, some have suggested replacing the Evans procedure with CCJ distraction arthrodesis with a laterally based bone graft.[6,7] However, this procedure decreases the mobility of the hindfoot, with isolated CCJ fusions decreasing range of motion at the talonavicular joint by 62% and at the subtalar joint by 30%.[8] The combination of a lateral column lengthening and an MDCO, commonly referred to as a double calcaneal osteotomy, allows for adduction of the midfoot and forefoot as well as increasing the supinatory force of the Achilles tendon by shifting its insertion site more medially.[9]

Two types of calcaneal Z osteotomies have been described in efforts to combine the desired effects of a double calcaneal osteotomy. The distal calcaneal Z osteotomy has been described by several investigators and incorporates the ability to translate and rotate the calcaneus just proximal to the CCJ (**Fig. 3**).[10–12] A more proximal calcaneal Z osteotomy was introduced by Malerba and DeMarchi,[13] which involved a lateral closing wedge resection for the treatment of hindfoot varus; this procedure was then modified by Weil and Roukis[14] to treat hindfoot valgus by shifting the posterior calcaneus medially and incorporating laterally based wedge grafts in the dorsal and/or plantar arms of the Z osteotomy.

In 1936, Cotton[15] first described an opening wedge osteotomy of the medial cuneiform for use in the flexible flatfoot deformity. He believed this type of osteotomy would

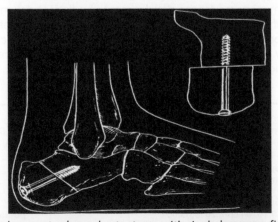

Fig. 1. Medial displacement calcaneal osteotomy with single lag screw fixation.

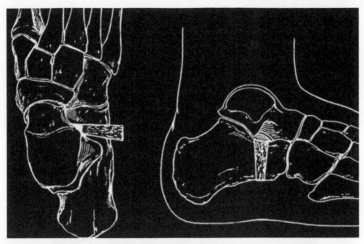

Fig. 2. Evans lateral column lengthening osteotomy.

restore the triangle of support of the static foot. The goal of this osteotomy is to preserve first ray mobility while providing a plantarflexory moment of the medial column in patients with residual fixed forefoot varus.

MEDIAL DISPLACEMENT CALCANEAL OSTEOTOMY

The traditional surgical approach for the MDCO is from the lateral aspect of the calcaneus. The patient is placed in a lateral decubitus position on the operating room table with general anesthesia and a regional nerve block. The incision is made on the lateral aspect of the heel posterior to the peroneal tendons and the sural nerve (**Fig. 4**). Sharp dissection is performed and the periosteum of the calcaneus is exposed (**Fig. 5**). Hohmann retractors are used both in the superior and inferior aspects of the incision to protect the Achilles and plantar fascia, respectively. A sagittal saw is used to perform the osteotomy from lateral to medial with the saw blade at 90° to the lateral wall of the calcaneus. Care should be used to protect the neurovascular and tendinous structures while completing the osteotomy on the medial side. If the saw blade courses too far on the medial aspect of the calcaneus, the toes often plantarflex. To protect the neurovascular structures, it is recommended to complete the osteotomy with a wide osteotome (**Fig. 6**). Once the osteotomy is completed, a lamina spreader is

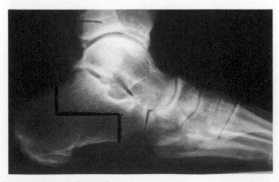

Fig. 3. Calcaneal Z osteotomy orientation.

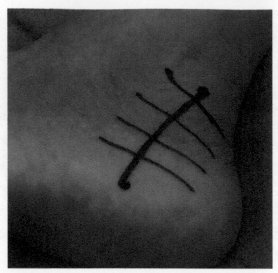

Fig. 4. Incision placement for the MDCO along the lateral calcaneus in an oblique manner posterior to the peroneal tendons and sural nerve.

used to distract the osteotomy to relax the soft-tissue attachments on the calcaneus to get a proper medial shift.

This osteotomy is purely a translational shift of the posterior tuberosity in the medial direction. It is recommended not to apply an additional varus force to the tuberosity during the medial shift. An intraoperative calcaneal axial view is helpful to ensure a vertical heel is obtained without creating an iatrogenic varus deformity (**Fig. 7**).

Fixation of the MDCO is done using Kirschner wires, staples, 1 or 2 lag screws, or a laterally based plate (**Fig. 8**). The MDCO often heals without minimal concerns of a

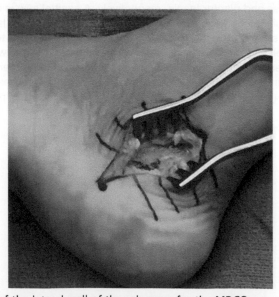

Fig. 5. Exposure of the lateral wall of the calcaneus for the MDCO.

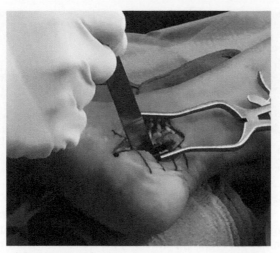

Fig. 6. Completion of the MDCO with a broad osteotome to protect the neurovascular structures on the medial aspect of the foot.

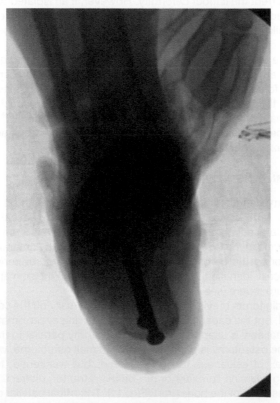

Fig. 7. Intraoperative calcaneal axial view of the MDCO demonstrating a pure medial shift of the posterior tuberosity of the calcaneus.

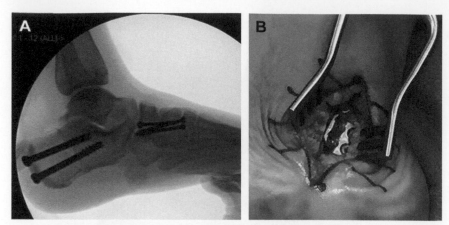

Fig. 8. (A) Fixation of the MDCO with 2 large cannulated lag screws. (B) Alternative fixation of the MDCO with a stepped locking plate along the lateral wall of the calcaneus.

nonunion. One study found an overall healing rate of 97% of MDCO with 3 different fixation methods.[16] This study also demonstrated a hardware removal rate of 47% of headed screws, 11% of headless screws, and 6% of lateral plates.

The postoperative course of this osteotomy is often dictated by the use of additional procedures to correct the flatfoot deformity. However, if an isolated osteotomy is performed, protected weight bearing in a cast can be performed at 3 weeks, with transition to a boot walker by the 6-week period or when consolidation of osteotomy is seen on radiographs.

The MDCO is a technically straightforward procedure used in stage II PTTD. It can be performed in any clinical situation when hindfoot valgus is present to convert the Achilles tendon force from a deforming valgus direction to an inverting one.[17] The MDCO protects the medial soft-tissue structures in flatfoot reconstruction, namely, the posterior tibial tendon and flexor digitorum longus tendon.[18,19] This osteotomy provides the necessary off-loading force to protect a repaired posterior tibial tendon or transferred flexor digitorum longus tendon.

LATERAL COLUMN LENGTHENING (EVANS OSTEOTOMY)

The lateral column lengthening procedure is achieved through an opening wedge osteotomy of the anterior calcaneus. Patient positioning is identical to what is used for an MDCO, lateral decubitus with general anesthesia. A 5- to 7-cm transverse incision is made starting at the CCJ, traveling proximally along the anterior calcaneus parallel and superior to the peroneal tendons (**Fig. 9**). The sural nerve and peroneal tendons are typically identified in the inferior aspect of the incision and are protected throughout the procedure (see **Fig. 9**).

The extensor digitorum brevis muscle is reflected dorsally off the calcaneus and the CCJ is identified, but the capsule is not violated. Starting approximately 13 mm from the CCJ, a sagittal saw is used to create the osteotomy parallel to the CCJ (**Fig. 10**). Completion of the osteotomy is performed with a small osteotome, which also allows the medial cortex of calcaneus to be preserved, but weakened, to obtain proper distraction. Using a lamina spreader or pin-based retractor, distraction of the osteotomy allows for insertion of the bone graft (**Fig. 11**). Tricortical patellar or iliac crest allograft has been the traditional form of bone graft for lateral column lengthening and is recommended by the authors (**Fig. 12**). However, new technology has now allowed

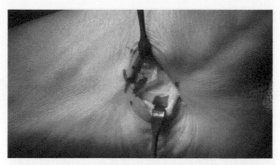

Fig. 9. Incision approach to the Evans lateral column lengthening starting at the calcaneo-cuboid joint and traveling proximally along the anterior calcaneus.

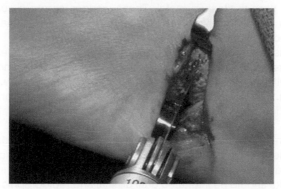

Fig. 10. A sagittal saw is used to perform the Evans osteotomy starting approximately 13 mm proximal from the calcaneocuboid joint.

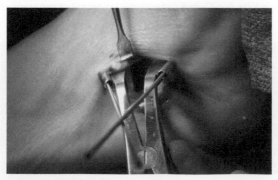

Fig. 11. A pin-based distractor can be placed across the osteotomy to facilitate distraction to fill with bone graft.

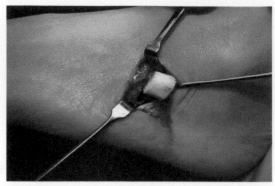

Fig. 12. Insertion of a tricortical iliac crest allograft wedge for distraction of the Evans osteotomy.

surgeons to choose from prefashioned, size-specific Evans wedges made of either allograft bone or porous titanium metal. These wedges create a custom length for distraction of the osteotomy, while also allowing the surgeon to dial in the amount of correction needed with trial sizing wedges before final insertion.

Fixation options to secure the bone graft have historically included no fixation or percutaneous Kirschner wires; however, most surgeons recommend at least some form of fixation with a small-diameter screw, low-profile locking plates, or an opening wedge plate (**Fig. 13**). Although it is reasonable not to fixate the graft, the authors recommend fixation to minimize displacement and micromotion at the graft-host interface.

Postoperative recovery course of an Evans osteotomy often includes 4 to 6 weeks of non–weight-bearing immobilization. Serial postoperative radiographs should monitor incorporation of the bone graft. Protected weight bearing in a boot walker from 6 to 10 weeks should be instituted until clinical and radiographic healing occurs. Although the incidence of a nonunion after the Evans osteotomy is low, care should be taken to ensure the osteotomy is fully healed before transitioning to regular shoegear.[20]

Lateral column lengthening is a powerful procedure that reconstructs the medial arch and corrects peritalar lateral subluxation. The clinical indication in stage II AAFD is a patient with a clinically reducible hindfoot with deformity in both the transverse and sagittal planes. DuMontier and colleagues[21] demonstrated the mechanism of flatfoot correction with the Evans osteotomy using a 3-dimensional flatfoot cadaver

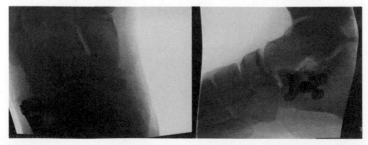

Fig. 13. Fixation of the Evans lateral column lengthening osteotomy with an opening wedge locking plate.

model. They demonstrated that, as the lateral column is lengthened, the midfoot is directed in an adducted and plantarflexed position relative to the hindfoot, which increases arch height with contributions from the long plantar ligament, plantar talonavicular capsule, and the lateral portion of the calcaneonavicular ligament. In addition, they did not show a varus movement of the calcaneus relative to the talus; however, clinically the foot is in a corrected position because the midfoot and forefoot are in a more anatomic alignment relative to the hindfoot.

CALCANEAL Z OSTEOTOMY (MALERBA, SCARF OSTEOTOMIES)

The calcaneal Z osteotomy is a useful procedure that combines the effects of both the MDCO and the Evans lateral column lengthening into one osteotomy. The surgical approach is similar to that described earlier, with the patient in a lateral decubitus position with general anesthesia. The incision is placed in a transverse manner over the anterior calcaneus; however, it is placed more proximally to incorporate the transverse and vertical arms (**Fig. 14**). The periosteum in incised, and the lateral wall of the calcaneus is exposed. Care should be taken to expose both the peroneal longus and brevis tendons, which should be retracted either superiorly or inferiorly during the completion of the osteotomy.

The osteotomy is created with 3 portions: (1) the posterior proximal arm exiting superiorly in the posterior tuberosity, (2) a transverse horizontal arm parallel to the plantar surface, and (3) the anterior inferior arm in the region of the traditional Evans osteotomy (see **Fig. 3**). These 3 arms of the osteotomy are ideally at right angles to each other. The osteotomy is performed with a sagittal saw starting with the posterior superior arm and ending with the anterior inferior arm. The osteotomy, which is through and through the calcaneus, is completed with an osteotome (**Fig. 15**).

The osteotomy is first shifted in a medial direction similar to an MDCO and pinned temporarily with 1 or 2 guidewires for cannulated lag screw fixation. Second, a pin-based distractor is placed in the anterior portion of the calcaneus to provide distraction of the anterior portion to accomplish lengthening of the lateral column (**Fig. 16**). Correction of the flatfoot deformity is then confirmed with intraoperative fluoroscopy, ensuring the talar head coverage has been corrected.

Insertion of bone graft into the anterior calcaneus is then performed before final fixation of the posterior calcaneal arm. Prefashioned allograft or titanium wedges can be placed in the anterior arm to hold distraction for the lateral column lengthening portion.

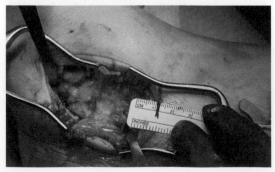

Fig. 14. Incision placement and approach to the calcaneal Z osteotomy. A transverse approach distally over the anterior calcaneus is made, while the proximal aspect is carried over the posterior tuberosity.

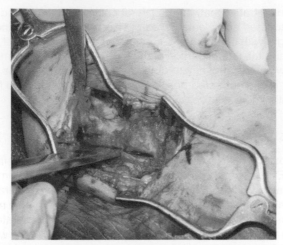

Fig. 15. Completion of the calcaneal Z osteotomy with an osteotome.

Next, fixation with 1 or 2 cannulated lag screws is delivered through the posterior proximal arm (**Figs. 17** and **18**). This fixation must be performed after placing the bone graft for the lateral column lengthening because the posterior arm must be semimobile to accommodate the insertion of the graft (Video 1).

   This osteotomy incorporates a wide bony surface area, which allows early consolidation and inherent stability. Protected weight bearing can usually be instituted with

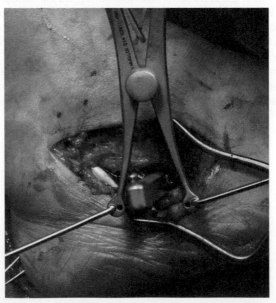

Fig. 16. A pin-based distractor is placed on the anterior-inferior arm of the Z osteotomy to facilitate lateral column lengthening. Insertion of an allograft or titanium wedge is then performed. In this figure, a trial size wedge is placed to confirm deformity correction.

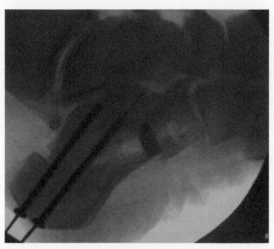

Fig. 17. Final fixation of the calcaneal Z osteotomy with 2 cannulated lag screws to fixate the proximal vertical arm and a titanium wedge to accomplish lateral column lengthening.

the calcaneal Z osteotomy at 6 to 8 weeks postoperation, depending on radiographic consolidation and the use of additional surgical procedures.

The calcaneal Z osteotomy is also a powerful procedure that can be used to replace the double calcaneal osteotomy (MDCO and Evans osteotomy). This osteotomy offers the benefits of both the MDCO and Evans osteotomy, allowing translation medially and lengthening of the lateral column. This osteotomy also provides 3-dimensional correction of the flexible abducted and valgus foot.

MEDIAL CUNEIFORM OPENING WEDGE OSTEOTOMY (COTTON OSTEOTOMY)

Forefoot supinatus is a commonly acquired soft-tissue adaption seen in AAFD in which the forefoot is inverted on the hindfoot.[22] Treatment of this clinical finding is achieved with a medial cuneiform opening wedge osteotomy, or Cotton osteotomy. The first ray must be reducible in order for this procedure to correct an elevated medial

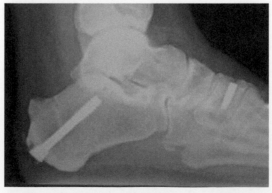

Fig. 18. Alternate fixation of the calcaneal Z osteotomy with a cannulated headless compression screw for the posterior vertical arm and an unfixated allograft wedge for lateral column lengthening.

column, and the first tarsometatarsal joint must also be free of degenerative joint disease.

The Cotton osteotomy is often performed last in flatfoot reconstruction. The patient is placed in a supine position under general anesthesia. A straight dorsal incision approximately 3 to 4 cm in length is placed over the medial cuneiform (**Fig. 19**). A periosteal incision is made, and the dorsal cortex is exposed. The first tarsometatarsal joint distally and the naviculocuneiform joint proximally should be identified, but the capsule and dorsal ligaments should not be violated to maintain stability of the osteotomy. The osteotomy is then planned in the dorsal, central aspect of the medial cuneiform with the assistance of lateral intraoperative fluoroscopy.

A sagittal saw is used to perform the osteotomy from dorsal to plantar. Care should be taken to avoid iatrogenic damage to the adjacent intermediate cuneiform or the second metatarsal by the saw blade. Completion of the osteotomy with an osteotome and lamina spreader allows distraction of the medial cuneiform and relaxation of the ligaments (**Fig. 20**). The plantar cortex should also be kept intact to provide proper plantarflexion of the first ray rather than pure lengthening if the plantar cortex is violated.

Once the amount of correction is achieved, bone graft is inserted in the osteotomy (**Fig. 21**). Similar to Evans osteotomy, numerous bone graft options are available, including autograft and allograft wedges. The authors prefer to use tricortical allograft iliac crest or porous titanium metal wedges. Because of the intrinsic stability of the osteotomy with the dorsal and plantar ligaments, fixation of the osteotomy is rarely performed. If needed, a Kirschner wire, dorsal plate, or staple may be used (**Figs. 22** and **23**). Postoperative course is similar to the Evans osteotomy with no weight

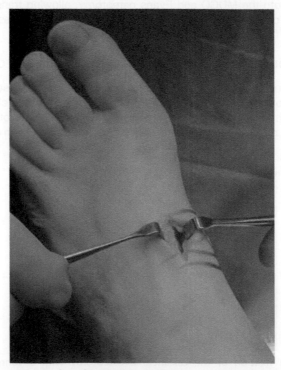

Fig. 19. Incision approach for the Cotton osteotomy straight dorsal over the medial cuneiform.

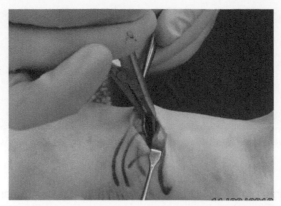

Fig. 20. A distractor or lamina spreader is used to distract the osteotomy before placing appropriate bone graft.

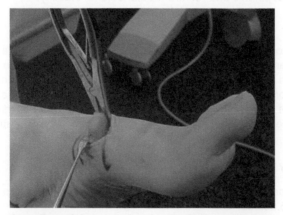

Fig. 21. Insertion of an allograft bone wedge for the Cotton osteotomy.

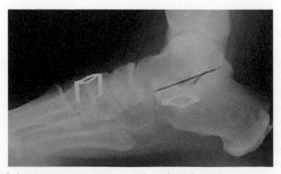

Fig. 22. Fixation of the Cotton osteotomy with a dorsal staple.

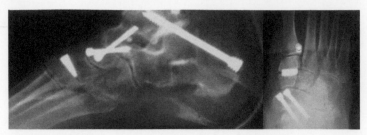

Fig. 23. Alternatively, insertion of a porous titanium wedge for Cotton osteotomy without fixation.

bearing for the first 4 to 6 weeks, followed by protected weight bearing in a walking boot at 6 weeks. Clinical and radiographic incorporation of the osteotomy dictates when to begin weight bearing after surgery.

Stabilization of the medial column is critical to success of flexible adult flatfoot reconstruction. If left untreated, forefoot supinatus can lead to lateral forefoot overload following calcaneal osteotomy. The Cotton osteotomy is an effective procedure to reduce forefoot supinatus and restore medial column stability.

SUMMARY

Flexible adult acquired flatfoot disorder is commonly treated with the use of osteotomies in the calcaneus and medial column. The combination of these joint-preserving osteotomies with additional soft-tissue procedures allows realignment of the hindfoot with the goal of preventing further deformity or degenerative joint disease. A thorough understanding of each patient's condition allows the surgeon to match the correct osteotomy to the clinical indication, while also successfully executing the planned surgery.

SUPPLEMENTARY DATA

Supplementary data related to this article can be found online at http://dx.doi.org/10.1016/j.cpm.2015.03.002.

REFERENCES

1. Lee MS, Vanore JV, Thomas JL, et al. Diagnosis and treatment of adult flatfoot. J Foot Ankle Surg 2005;44:78–113.
2. Johnson KA, Strom DE. Tibialis posterior tendon dysfunction. Clin Orthop Relat Res 1989;(239):196–206.
3. Gleich A. Beitzagzur operativen plattsfussbehandlung. Arch Klin Chir 1893;46:358–62.
4. Koutsogiannis E. Treatment of mobile flat foot by displacement osteotomy of the calcaneus. J Bone Joint Surg Br 1971;53B:96–100.
5. Evans D. Calcaneovalgus deformity. J Bone Joint Surg Br 1975;57:270–8.
6. Haeseker GA, Mureau MA, Faber FW. Lateral column lengthening for the acquired adult flatfoot deformity caused by posterior tibial tendon dysfunction stage II: a retrospective comparison of calcaneus osteotomy with calcaneocuboid distraction arthrodesis. J Foot Ankle Surg 2010;49(4):380–4.
7. van der Krans A, Louwerens JW, Anderson P. Adult acquired flexible flatfoot, treated by calcaneocuboid distraction arthrodesis, posterior tibial tendon

augmentation, and percutaneous Achilles tendon lengthening: a prospective outcome study of 20 patients. Acta Orthop 2006;77(1):156–63.

8. Deland JT, Otis JC, Lee KT, et al. Lateral column lengthening with calcaneocuboid fusion: range of motion in the triple joint complex. Foot Ankle Int 1995; 16(11):729–33.

9. Catanzariti AR, Mendicino RW, King GL, et al. Double calcaneal osteotomy: realignment considerations in eight patients. J Am Podiatr Med Assoc 2005; 95(1):53–9.

10. Griend RV. Lateral column lengthening using a "Z" osteotomy of the calcaneus. Tech Foot Ankle Surg 2008;7(4):257–63.

11. Knupp M, Horisberger M, Hintermann B. A new Z-shaped calcaneal osteotomy for 3-plane correction of severe varus deformity of the hindfoot. Tech Foot Ankle Surg 2008;7(2):90–5.

12. Scott RT, Berlet GC. Calcaneal Z osteotomy for extra-articular correction of hindfoot valgus. J Foot Ankle Surg 2013;52(3):406–8.

13. Malerba F, De Marchi F. Calcaneal osteotomies. Foot Ankle Clin 2005;10(3): 523–40.

14. Weil LS Jr, Roukis TS. The calcaneal scarf osteotomy: operative technique. J Foot Ankle Surg 2001;40(3):178–82.

15. Cotton FJ. Foot statics and surgery. N Engl J Med 1936;214:353–62.

16. Abbasian A, Zaidi R, Guha A, et al. Comparison of three different fixation methods of calcaneal osteotomies. Foot Ankle Int 2013;34:420–5.

17. Trnka HJ, Easley ME, Myerson MS. The role of calcaneal osteotomies for correction of adult flatfoot. Clin Orthop Relat Res 1999;365:50–64.

18. Sung IH, Lee S, Otis JC, et al. Posterior tibial tendon force requirement in early heel rise after calcaneal osteotomies. Foot Ankle Int 2002;23:842–9.

19. Guha AR, Perera AM. Calcaneal osteotomy in the treatment of adult acquired flatfoot deformity. Foot Ankle Clin N Am 2012;17:247–58.

20. Prissel MA, Roukis TS. Incidence of nonunion of the unfixated, isolated Evans calcaneal osteotomy: a systematic review. J Foot Ankle Surg 2012;51:323–5.

21. DuMontier TA, Falicov A, Mosca V, et al. Calcaneal lengthening: investigation of deformity correction in a cadaver flatfoot model. Foot Ankle Int 2005;26(2): 166–70.

22. Evans EL, Catanzariti AR. Forefoot supinatus. Clin Podiatr Med Surg 2014;31: 405–13.

Osteotomies for the Management of Charcot Neuroarthropathy of the Foot and Ankle

(R) CrossMark

Ryan T. Scott, DPM, FACFAS[a],*, William T. DeCarbo, DPM, FACFAS[b],
Christopher F. Hyer, DPM, MS, FACFAS[c]

KEYWORDS

• Charcot • Midfoot osteotomy • External fixation

KEY POINTS

• Charcot neuroarthropathy is often devastating to the structure and stability of the foot and ankle.
• This disease may require permanent bracing, reconstructive surgical stabilization, and in some cases lower leg amputation.
• Successful management of Charcot requires diligence and surveillance by physician and patient alike.

PRESENTATION

Patients with diabetic neuropathy that develop unstable Charcot neuroarthropathy not only have an autoimmune disease that prolongs the healing process, they also often have an inability to maintain a non–weight bearing status. The presence of the autoimmune disease and hyperglycemia impair the inflammatory response blunting the delivery of growth factors essential for wound healing. This same lack of inflammatory response leads to decreased bone callous formation in the presence of increased osteoclastic activity.[1] Patients with diabetes and neuropathy often have balance difficulties with lack of coordination, weak upper body strength, and an overall body habitus not amenable to strict non–weight bearing.

Charcot typically presents with hallmark signs of a red, hot, swollen foot with bounding pulses.[2] Pain may or may not be present because of the severity of

Disclosure: No commercial or financial conflicts of interest.
[a] Department of Orthopedics, The CORE Institute, 18444 N 25th Avenue, Unit 320, Phoenix, AZ 85023, USA; [b] The Orthopedic Group, Pittsburgh, PA, USA; [c] Orthopedic Foot and Ankle Center, Westerville Medical Campus, 300 Polaris Parkway, Suite 2000, Westerville, OH 43082, USA
* Corresponding author.
E-mail address: scottryt@gmail.com

Clin Podiatr Med Surg 32 (2015) 405–418
http://dx.doi.org/10.1016/j.cpm.2015.03.004
0891-8422/15/$ – see front matter © 2015 Elsevier Inc. All rights reserved.

peripheral neuropathy in these patients. The patient typically denies any history of remote trauma or significant event leading to the early presentation of Charcot. It is not uncommon for acute Charcot to be misdiagnosed as cellulitis, deep infection, or gouty arthritis. Clinically, early signs of deformity of the foot and ankle may be present. Hypermobility and crepitus is typically identified in the zone of involvement. In cases of Charcot with subsequent joint subluxation, an associated ulceration is often present medial-lateral depending on the bony prominence. Acute infection or chronic osteomyelitis can be present in the long-standing Charcot foot (**Table 1**).

ANATOMIC CLASSIFICATION (BRODSKY)
Type 1: Midfoot

The midfoot is the most common zone of occurrence (60%), typically involving the tatarsometatarsal and talonavicular joints.[3] These joints are often stable but mal positioned leading to bony prominences and possible pressure ulceration.

Type 2: Hindfoot

The hindfoot is the second most common zone (35%), usually involving the subtalar, talonavicular, and calcanealcuboid joints. This zone is often extremely unstable leading to destructive deformity. Unfortunately, the instability may drive more proximal breakdown in the ankle. Zone 2 Charcot is often slow to consolidate leading to a longer non–weight bearing period.

Type 3: Ankle and Calcaneus

The least common of the three zones (5%) involves the ankle and calcaneus. There is devastating deformity, which has a tendency to break down extremely quickly because of the high stress of axial load. Charcot of the ankle and/or calcaneus is often limb-threatening. Significant instability, swelling, and ulceration are present (**Fig. 1**).

GOALS OF TREATMENT

There are many goals in the management of a patient with Charcot of the foot or ankle. Conservative and surgical management is often warranted depending the stage and severity. The ultimate goal is to obtain a plantar-grade foot that can later be braced or placed back into a shoe.[3]

Table 1 Classification of Charcot		
	Eichenholtz	
Grade 0		Joint edema Negative bone scan and radiographs
Grade 1	Fragmentation	Joint edema Radiographs show osseous fragmentation with joint dislocation
Grade 2	Coalescence	Decreased local edema Radiographs show coalescence of fragments and absorption of debris
Grade 3	Reconstruction	No local edema Radiographs show consolidation and remodeling of fracture fragments

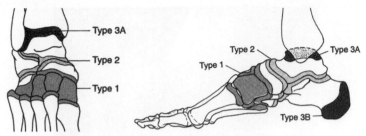

Fig. 1. Brodsky classification. (*From* Brodsky JW. The diabetic foot. In: Coughlin MJ, Mann RA, editors. Surgery of the foot and ankle. 8th edition. Philadelphia (PA): Mosby; 2007. p. 1341; with permission.)

Conservative Management

Conservative management is an appropriate option during the early onset of Charcot. The goal is to immediately place the patient non–weight bearing for an extended duration, often 3 to 4 months until quiescent stage is present. Multiple types of immobilization have been well described in the literature as effective means. However, the gold standard remains a total contact cast. Myerson and coworkers[4] originally described an efficacy of 75% offloading while using a total contact cast (TCC).

Unfortunately, many cases of Charcot do not present in the acute phase and often patients continue to weight-bear unaware of the destruction they are causing.

Surgical Management

Even with appropriate conservative care, most patients who undergo a Charcot event require some sort of surgical procedure. Surgical management may be indicated in 25% to 50% of patients with Charcot.[5] This is because of the destructive change in the architecture of the foot and ankle. Increased pressure and bony prominences lead to high-pressure areas and ultimately ulceration. The goals of Charcot reconstruction include restoration of alignment and stability, prevention of recurrence of ulceration, and prevention of amputation. The ultimate goal is to re-establish the foot to be braceable for supportive shoe gear and not necessarily restoration back to a normal foot.[6–12] A multitude of surgical procedures has shown results in the management of Charcot using internal fixation, external fixation, or a combination of both.

Multiple factors are considered when choosing fixation in this patient population including severity of the deformity, if an ulcer or infection is present, and acute or chronic osteomyelitis. In the presence of a large ulceration or acute osteomyelitis, which may compromise wound closure surgically, staged surgery is often used (**Fig. 2**). Once the ulcer is amenable to wound closure or the acute osteomyelitis is treated, definitive surgical reconstruction can be considered. In the presence of an ulcer that is not acutely infected, surgical correction of the deformity is often required for the soft tissue envelope to heal.

Timing of Surgery

Typically, surgical management of the Charcot foot and ankle was deferred until after completion of consolidation or Eichenholtz stage III.[13,14] The demineralization, soft bone, and swelling in stage I may increase technical difficulty and surgical complications, such as infection and loss of fixation.[5,13,14] Bone fragmentation may be a contraindication to surgery, and surgery is delayed until skin wrinkling has occurred.[4] The

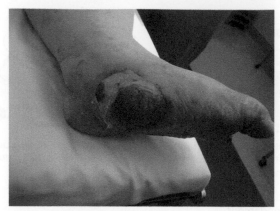

Fig. 2. Preoperative ulcer limiting soft tissue coverage.

specific selection criteria for those cases most likely to benefit from operative reduction during stage I remain the subject of discussion. Patient compliance with postoperative non–weight bearing may be important to the success of arthrodesis.[5]

Ostectomy

Typically, ostectomy is a simple surgical procedure with the least surgical risk. This procedure is typically selected when an ulceration or callus is present with a profound plantar bony prominence. Other indications include, but are not limited to, the elderly, sedentary inactive patients, and patients with a stable deformity. Typically, excision of the ulceration and primary closure is performed at the same time as the exostectomy. One of the greatest advantages of the exostectomy is rapid return to shoe gear and activity. Unfortunately, progressive recurrence of the ulceration and possible instability may occur.

Pinzur and colleagues[15] noted results at 3.6 years follow-up with 22 patients with Charcot and chronic open wounds. A total of 32 surgical procedures were performed, 16 underwent debridement of the infected bone and surrounding soft tissues, eight exostectomy, and seven partial excision of the deformed midfoot with arthrodesis. All surgical patients were managed postoperatively with long-term custom accommodative bracing. They found that most of the patients treated were able to remain ambulatory postoperatively. Five amputations were performed, three at the Syme ankle disarticulation level, one at the Chopart hindfoot level, and one at the midfoot level. None of the patients went on to require below-knee amputation.

Medially Based Midfoot Osteotomy

The medially based midfoot osteotomy is multifaceted in the correction of the midfoot and forefoot. This osteotomy allows for correction mostly in the sagittal and transverse planes. This osteotomy is typically used in the severe Charcot deformity involving multiple joints of the midfoot (**Fig. 3**).

The patient is placed supine with a bump under the ipsilateral hip bringing the foot to neutral. The leg is usually prepared to the knee to allow for the possibility of external fixation application. A medial incision is made along the medial column centrally located over the apex of the deformity. The incision is kept as full thickness as possible. The dorsal and plantar soft tissues are mobilized and retracted. We recommend the use of a wide Cobb elevator to release the soft tissue. Once adequate

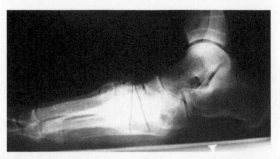

Fig. 3. Radiographic planning of triplanal midfoot osteotomy.

dissection is performed, two Steinmann pins are inserted from medial to lateral under fluoroscopic guidance encompassing the apex of the deformity. The authors routinely use 2-mm Steinmann pins as cutting guides (**Fig. 4**). The osteotomy is then created from medial to lateral in a triangular fashion with the apex dorsally. This osteotomy allows for closure on the medial side and a plantar flexion force when the osteotomy is fixated (**Fig. 5**). A second lateral incision is often created over the cuboid to aid in the removal of the resected bone. Fixation is at the discretion of the surgeon. We typically use large-diameter beam screws or bolts medially followed by plate fixation across the midfoot. The beam screws may be placed from distal to proximal or proximal to distal based on the comfort level of the surgeon. A large-bore screw (6.5 mm or larger) is recommended. A long thick locking plate with multiple screw trajectories and orientation seems to work best avoiding the beam screw when applied medially. It is important to capture the solid cortical and cancellous bone of the lateral column. Other fixation options include centrally and laterally based beam screws (**Fig. 6**). External fixation is often associated with this type of osteotomy because of the extent of osseous resection encompassing the entire midfoot. In cases of beam screw and no plate fixation, the "bent wire" compression can be used with a fine wire external fixator.

Charcot of the Ankle

When thinking about Charcot, one typically thinks of the midfoot and forefoot as the major culprit, not necessarily the ankle. Charcot of the ankle is usually viewed as more of a limb-threatening disorder when compared with the foot. Deformity of the ankle usually results in a varus or valgus deformity leading to increasing pressure to

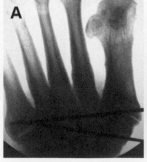
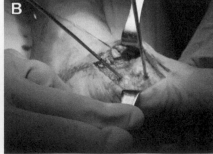

Fig. 4. (*A, B*) Use of Steinmann pins as a cutting template.

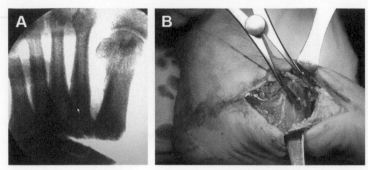

Fig. 5. (*A, B*) Resection of bone from medial to lateral allowing for closure of the abduction deformity.

the hindfoot, midfoot, and forefoot. Appropriate weight-bearing radiographs are crucial in identifying the center of rotational axis for the osteotomy.

When Charcot of the ankle occurs, the talus is typically involved. This can lead to loss of stability of the ankle in a global-type fashion encompassing the medial and lateral tibiotalar joint. Often, there is fracture and fragmentation of the talus leading to a nonsalvageable tibiotalar joint. This raises the use of hindfoot arthrodesis nails, femoral head allografts, and large robust plating. TTC, tibiocalcaneal, tibiotalar, and subtalar arthrodesis are the routine arthrodesis typically performed. If the talus is salvageable, the use of a hindfoot nail for a TTC is recommended because of load sharing and static/dynamic capabilities. Often external fixation is used on conjunction over the intramedullary nail (**Fig. 7**). Similarly, when the talus is not salvageable, a tibio-calcaneal arthrodesis or femoral head allograft is used with a similar construct. We typically prefer the use of the calcar of the femoral head allograft because of its cortical strength. The actual femoral head can then be sacrificed for cancellous chips for void filler around the planned fusion site. The largest benefit of the femoral head allograft is to act like a spacer to help maintain limb length.

Arthrodesis

Arthrodesis of the involved joints is the gold standard in the management of the Charcot foot and ankle.[5,16] Isolated or multiple level arthrodesis is typically performed in conjunction with other procedures. Talonavicular and naviculocuneiform joint arthrodesis are the more commonly performed isolated joint fusions of the midfoot.

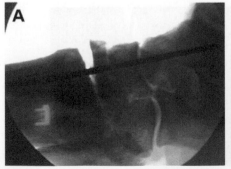
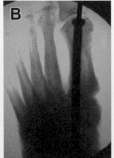
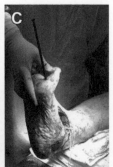

Fig. 6. (*A–C*) Beaming of the medial column.

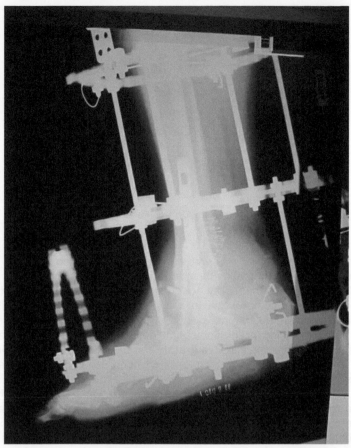

Fig. 7. Intramedullary nail with external fixation. Note proximal tibial ring distance from nail.

Isolated procedures are often very powerful when performed correctly at the unstable midfoot joint. Adequate joint preparation down to good healthy bleeding cancellous bone is absolutely necessary. Often autograft or allograft may be warranted to aid in arthrodesis. Larger cannulated screws (5.0 mm) with the addition of locking plates are sufficient. LaPorta and colleagues[17] recently presented a case series on TTC arthrodesis in the Charcot population with the use of internal and external fixation in combination. They concluded that in the patient with Charcot neuroarthropathy without osteomyelitis, the concomitant use of external fixation and internal fixation further stabilizes the deformed, neuropathic, high-risk foot. The frame neutralizes stress at the arthrodesis site until the bone has consolidated.

External Fixation Augmentation

External fixation is advantageous in patients with poor soft tissue envelopes, large bone defects, peripheral arterial disease, and current or previous infections of the soft tissue or bone (**Fig. 8**). External fixation also allows continued and immediate weight bearing to patients not able to remain non–weight bearing or in patients with a history of deep venous thrombosis or comorbidities increasing patient risk for

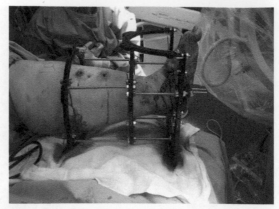

Fig. 8. Staged reconstruction with medial skin healed.

deep venous thrombosis. Patients with diabetic Charcot often lack the ability to remain non–weight bearing, putting them at risk for falls and further injury.

External fixators have the ability to correct deformities while simultaneously providing stability and compression to a fusion site. Rigidity and stability of the construct is provided through transosseous wires or pins, which are not dependent of cortical purpose making this fixation option ideal in this patient population. Various constructs of multiplanar ring and wire fixators can be used for static fixation, stabilization to off-load a deformity or ulcer, or used for dynamic correction of deformities.[18–21]

In Charcot reconstructions static circular external fixation is used primarily for stability or to augment internal fixation. These frames are usually prebuilt for ease of application. The construct usually consists of a tibial block, consisting of two circular tibial rings, attached to a footplate (**Fig. 9**). This construct allows stabilization of the ankle, hindfoot, and midfoot. In the absence of acute or chronic soft tissue or bone infection this is the authors' primary application of external fixation. The external fixation is applied after an acute corrective osteotomy with rigid internal fixation. This allows maintenance of the correction and weight bearing as tolerated (**Fig. 10**). This

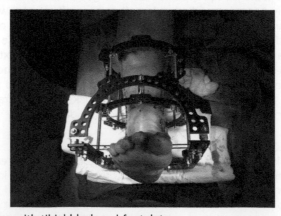

Fig. 9. Static frame with tibial block and footplate.

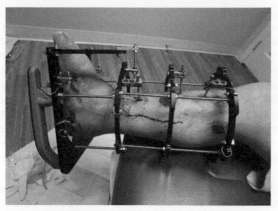

Fig. 10. Footplate for weight bearing.

combined fixation improves mechanical stability and controls surrounding joints through the healing process. When combining fixation attention to preoperative surgical planning is imperative so that enough space is maintained to provide both techniques. Often with medial column plating transosseous wires through the midfoot are challenging to place. The same concept applies when combined with an intramedullary rod and external fixation. Careful attention is needed to maintain an adequate bone bridge between the tip of the rod and any transosseous fixation to the external fixator. Lack of an adequate bone bridge may cause a stress riser leading to fracture.

In the absence of internal fixation this same static circular construct can provide stability and compression through a corrective osteotomy. For midfoot or hindfoot Charcot a "bent wire" technique is used for compression. The tibial block is applied the same way in either application. For midfoot osteotomy compression and stability temporary fixation with Steinmann pins is used to reduce the osteotomy (**Fig. 11**). The calcaneus is attached to the footplate in the normal fashion. A transosseous smooth wire is placed through the metatarsals distal to the osteotomy. This wire is then

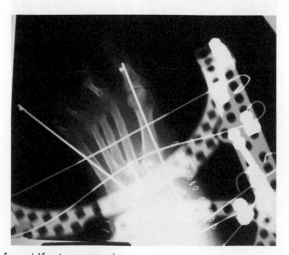

Fig. 11. Arc wire for midfoot compression.

"walked" proximal on the footplate and attached creating an arc in the wire with the concavity toward the osteotomy. Once the wire is tensioned the arc flattens out creating compression through the osteotomy site. At this point the temporary Steinmann pins used to maintain the correction can be removed or left in for the duration of the treatment per the surgeons' preference. If compression is required through the subtalar joint a smooth wire is place through the talar neck. This wire is arced inferiorly and proximally and attached to the footplate. Again, once tensioned the arc flattens out causing compression (**Fig. 12**). For compression through the ankle joint the static frame is attached as previously described. Compression is achieved by pressing the footplate to the tibial block through the threaded rods of the external fixator. As with the midfoot, temporary Steinmann pins can be used to obtain correction while the fixator is applied and compressed. These pins can also be maintained through the correction if desired. If the choice is made to maintain the pins they can be either bent to remain external to the plantar heel or bent and buried to the calcaneal bone for later removal (**Figs. 13** and **14**). Pinzur and colleagues[21] reported acute correction of Charcot neuroarthropathy with a static external fixation in patients with osteomyelitis. A total of 68 of the 71 patients (95.7%) achieved limb salvage and were able to ambulate in commercial therapeutic footwear with this technique.

Dynamic correction is sometimes used in this patient population to obtain gradual correction. The most common indications are for patients that are high risk in regard to neurovascular injury or have major soft tissue compromise. The traditional Ilizarov technique with multiple hinges and motors or the Taylor Spatial Frame (Smith & Nephew, Memphis, TN, USA) for concomitant correction in all three cardinal body

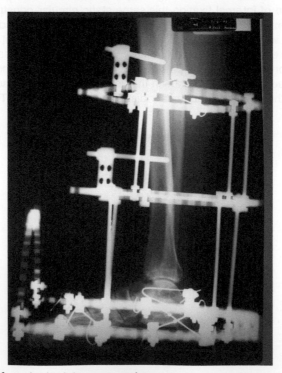

Fig. 12. Arc wire for subtalar joint compression.

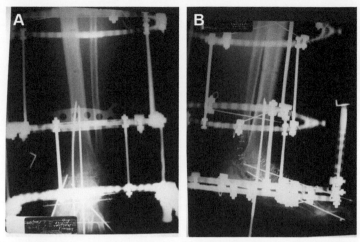

Fig. 13. (*A, B*) Staged reconstruction once wound is healed with external fixation and percutaneous Steinmann pins.

planes is used. In the authors' opinion gradual correction has less application because of the amount of diseased bone that is usually present in Charcot patients with diabetes. Once all the infected or nonviable bone is resected the foot or ankle is usually decompressed enough where an acute correction can be made under no skin or soft tissue tension.

Maintenance of the external fixator in the patient population is usually about 3 months. Several factors dictate this timeline including patient comorbidities, if a combination of internal or external fixation was used, and evidence of osseous union. At times when combined fixation is used the external fixator may be removed sooner because internal stabilization is present. This is patient dependent. In some cases with suspected osteomyelitis, bone cultures are taken at the time of the initial surgery. The surgical correction and compression is maintained with the external fixator as described. If the bone cultures are negative, percutaneous internal fixation can be used when the external fixator is removed (**Fig. 15**).

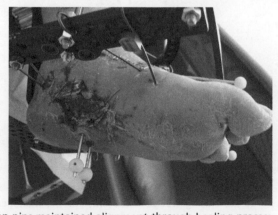

Fig. 14. Steinmann pins maintained alignment through healing process.

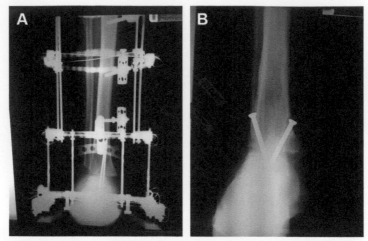

Fig. 15. (*A, B*) Percutaneous screws with removal of external fixation and negative bone cultures.

REHABILITATION AND RECOVERY

Rehabilitation of Charcot is multifactorial. The overall health and well-being of the patient is critical in the outcome of the surgical procedures. Ensuring appropriate blood sugar control and adequate protein intake helps reduce the risk of delayed healing of the surgical wounds and ulcerations. Patient compliance with a non–weight bearing status for the first 6 to 8 weeks is essential. Local wound care of the ulceration and pin care around the external fixation wires increase the overall success of the surgical reconstruction. If an external fixator is used, it is removed 8 weeks postoperatively.

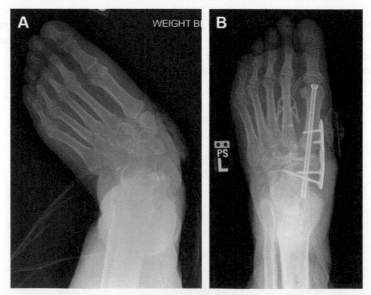

Fig. 16. (*A, B*) Power of the closing wedge osteotomy for the management of Charcot neuroarthropathy.

The patient then is placed into a weight-bearing cast for 3 weeks. In patients not placed into an external fixator we prefer to place these patients into a removable cast or cam boot around Week 8 pending the need for wound care. This allows for appropriate initiation of physical therapy. These patients then are allowed to weight bear in their walking boot for 3 weeks. Serial radiographs are used to help determine advancement to a full weight-bearing status in regular shoe gear or bracing.

SUMMARY

In conclusion, Charcot neuroarthropathy is often devastating to the structure and stability of the foot and ankle. This disease may require permanent bracing, reconstructive surgical stabilization, and in some cases lower leg amputation. Successful management of Charcot requires diligence and surveillance by physician and patient (Fig. 16).

REFERENCES

1. Stapleton JJ, Zgonis T. Surgical reconstruction of the diabetic Charcot foot. Clin Podiatr Med Surg 2012;29:425–33.
2. Varma AK. Charcot neuroarthropathy of the foot and ankle: a review. J Foot Ankle Surg 2013;52(6):740–9.
3. Brodsky JW. The diabetic foot. In: Coughlin MJ, Mann RA, editors. Surgery of the foot and Ankle. 7th edition. St Louis (MO): Mosby; 1999. p. 895–969.
4. Myerson MS, Henderson MR, Saxby T, et al. Management of midfoot diabetic neuroarthropathy. Foot Ankle Int 1994;15:233–41.
5. Trepman E, Nihal A, Pinzur M. Current topics review: Charcot neuroarthropathy of the foot and ankle. Foot Ankle Int 2005;26(1):26–46.
6. Zgonis T, Stapleton JJ, Jeffries LC, et al. Surgical treatment of Charcot neuroarthropathy. AORN J 2008;87:971–89.
7. Caravaggi C, Cimmino M, Caruso S, et al. Intramedullary compressive nail fixation for the treatment of severe Charcot deformity of the ankle and rear foot. J Foot Ankle Surg 2006;45:20–4.
8. Cinar M, Derincek A, Akpinar S. Tibiocalcaneal arthrodesis with posterior blade plate in diabetic neuroarthropathy. Foot Ankle Int 2010;32:511–6.
9. Fabrin J, Larsen K, Holstein PE. Arthrodesis with external fixation in the unstable or misaligned Charcot ankle in patients with diabetes mellitus. Int J Low Extrem Wounds 2007;6:102–7.
10. Jolly GP, Zgonis T, Polyzois V. External fixation in the management of Charcot neuroarthropathy. Clin Podiatr Med Surg 2003;20:741–56.
11. Pakarinen TK, Laine HJ, Honkonen SE, et al. Charcot arthropathy of the diabetic foot: current concepts and review of 36 cases. Scand J Surg 2002;91:195–201.
12. Yakacki CM, Gall K, Dirschl DR, et al. Pseudoelastic intramedullary nailing for tibio-talo-calcaneal arthrodesis. Expert Rev Med Devices 2001;8:159–66.
13. Eichenholtz SN. Charcot joints. Springfield (IL): Charles C Thomas; 1966.
14. Johnson JE. Operative treatment of neuropathic arthropathy of the foot and ankle. J Bone Joint Surg 1998;80-A:1700–9.
15. Pinzur M, Sage R, Stuck R, et al. A treatment algorithm for neuropathic (Charcot) midfoot deformity. Foot Ankle Int 1993;14(4):189–97.
16. Schon LC, Easley ME, Weinfield SB. Charcot neuroarthropathy of the foot and ankle. Clin Orthop Relat Res 1998;349:116–31.

17. LaPorta GA, Nasser EN, Mulhern JL. Tibiocalcaneal arthrodesis in the high-risk foot. J Foot Ankle Surg 2014;53:774–86. Available at: http://www.jfas.org/article/S1067-2516(14)00314-7/pdf.

18. Stapleton JJ, Belczyk R, Zgonis T. Revisional Charcot foot and ankle surgery. Clin Podiatr Med Surg 2009;26:127–39.

19. Capobianco DM, Stapleton JJ, Zgonis T. The role of an extended medial column arthrodesis for Charcot midfoot neuroarthropathy. Diabet Foot Ankle 2010;1. http://dx.doi.org/10.3402/dfa.v1i0.5282.

20. Facaros Z, Ramanujam CL, Stapleton JJ. Combined circular external fixation and open reduction internal fixation with pro-syndesmotic screws for repair of a diabetic ankle fracture. Diabet Foot Ankle 2010;1. http://dx.doi.org/10.3402/dfa.v1i0.5554.

21. Pinzur MS, Gil J, Belmares J. Treatment of osteomyelitis in Charcot foot with single-stage resection of infection, correction of deformity and maintenance with ring fixation. Foot Ankle Int 2012;33(12):1069–74.

Minimally Invasive Surgery Osteotomy of the Hindfoot

Joel Vernois, MD[a],*, David Redfern, FRCS(Tr&Orth)[b], Linda Ferraz, MD[c], Julien Laborde, MD[d]

KEYWORDS

- Minimally invasive surgery • Percutaneous surgery • Heel osteotomy
- Zadek osteotomy • Haglund • Calcaneoplasty

KEY POINTS

- Percutaneous surgery minimises soft tissue injury and preserves the soft tissue envelope.
- Percutaneous surgery offers a more versatile range of surgical options.
- The technique requires specific instruments, including a burr such as a 'Wedge' or a 'Shannon'.
- The procedures are reproducible with specific stepwise approach.
- Excellent anatomical knowledge essential to ensure minimum of risk.
- The techniques involve new technology and specific training is necessary to avoid complications.

PERCUTANEOUS CALCANEAL OSTEOTOMY
Medial Heel Shift

Introduction

Calcaneal osteotomy is a common and powerful procedure to correct varus or valgus of the hindfoot. The classic lateral approach is well known but complications have been described. Surgeons have tried to minimize scarring to avoid cutaneous complications. We have been performing percutaneous calcaneal osteotomy for the last 4 years. The procedure is performed under radiographic control and is a safe and efficient technique.

Technique

The procedure is performed with the patient lying in a lateral position (**Fig. 1**) or supine with a sandbag under the homolateral hip (**Fig. 2**). The operative foot is on top and is placed over the end of the table (see **Figs. 1** and **2**).

The authors have nothing to disclose.
[a] Sussex Orthopaedic NHS Treatment Center, Lewes Road, Haywards Heath RH16 4EY, West Sussex, UK; [b] London Foot and Ankle Centre, Hospital of St John and St Elizabeth, 60 Grove End Road, London NW8 9NH, UK; [c] 150 street Louis Landi, Nimes 30000, France; [d] Clinique de l'union, Boulevard Ratalens, Saint Jean 31240, France
* Corresponding author. 712 rue jean choquet, Picquigny 80310, France.
E-mail address: joel.vernois@sfr.fr

Clin Podiatr Med Surg 32 (2015) 419–434
http://dx.doi.org/10.1016/j.cpm.2015.03.008   podiatric.theclinics.com
0891-8422/15/$ – see front matter © 2015 Elsevier Inc. All rights reserved.

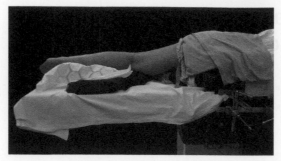

Fig. 1. The patient in a lateral position with the operative foot on top over the end of the table.

The C-arm is positioned underneath (**Fig. 3**). A thigh tourniquet is positioned. A popliteal block or spinal or general anesthesia is necessary.

The technique requires a Shannon burr 3 mm wide and 20 mm long, a specific burr driver with high torque and low speed, and a pencil driver (**Fig. 4**).

The osteotomy is first drawn on the lateral side of the heel. The apex of the chevron is located with a Kirschner wire (K-wire) and marked under radiography (**Fig. 5**). The superior and plantar cuts are landmarked on the skin to help the procedure (**Fig. 6**).

At the level of the apex, a short skin incision (6–7 mm) is made. The soft tissue is dissected with a Halsted until contact is made with the bone. The clip is kept open to prevent nerve lesion until the burr is totally introduced in to the bone (**Fig. 7**).

The osteotomy is performed at the speed of 350 rpm. Because of the width of the os calcis and the length of the burr, the osteotomy cannot be completed in 1 swipe. The lateral superior cortex is cut first (**Fig. 8**) and then used as a guide for the medial side. Regular fluoroscopy is performed to control the osteotomy. The inferior cut is performed with similar steps (**Fig. 9**).

As soon as the osteotomy is completed, the mobilization of the heel is checked. The translation is performed using a 2-mm K-wire introduced by the portal in the anterior part of the heel or a small periosteal elevator (**Fig. 10**). Used as a lever arm, the K-wire allows shifting medially and rotation of the posterior part of the calcaneus (**Fig. 11**). Once the correction is achieved, the osteotomy is fixed with 1 or 2 screws (≥6 mm) (**Figs. 12** and **13**).

The wound is closed with an absorbable suture.

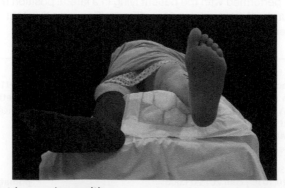

Fig. 2. The patient in a supine position.

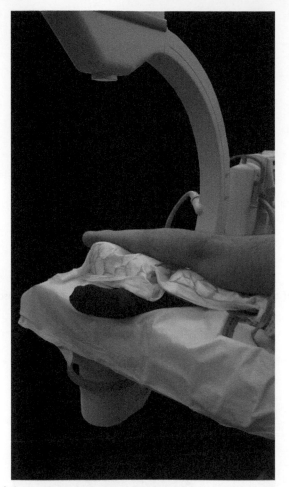

Fig. 3. Position of the C-arm.

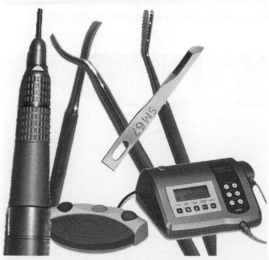

Fig. 4. Indispensable instruments: a burr 3 mm wide and 20 mm long, a specific burr driver, and a pencil driver.

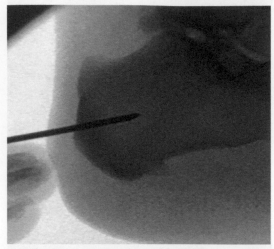

Fig. 5. Control of the position of the apex of the osteotomy with fluoroscopy.

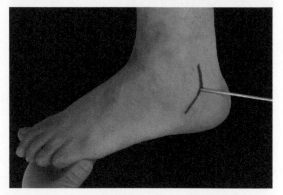

Fig. 6. The landmarks of the osteotomy are drawn on the skin.

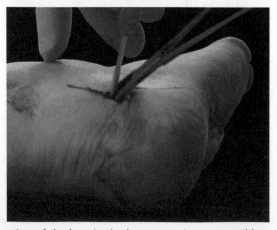

Fig. 7. The introduction of the burr in the bone must be protected by a clip.

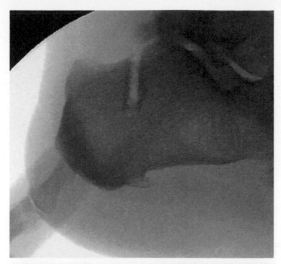

Fig. 8. The dorsal cut.

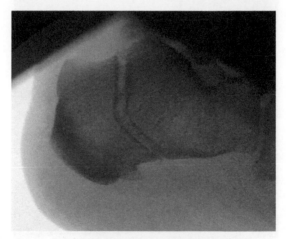

Fig. 9. The plantar cut.

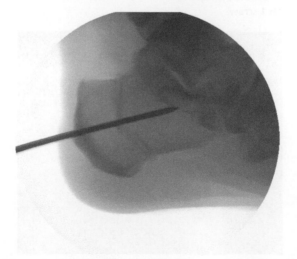

Fig. 10. Translation of the osteotomy. Lateral view.

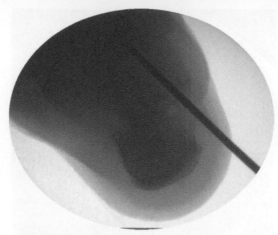

Fig. 11. Rotation and translation.

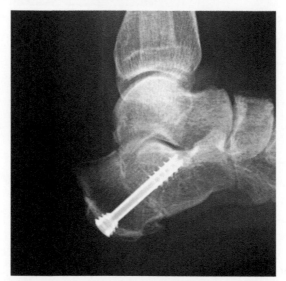

Fig. 12. Fixation with 1 screw.

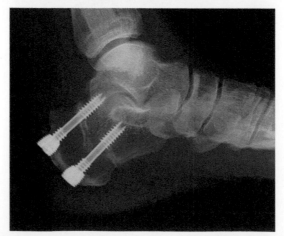

Fig. 13. Fixation with 2 screws.

Postoperative care

Depending on the additional procedures, an isolated heel osteotomy is immobilized with a walking boot for 2 months. Partial weight bearing with crutches is permitted depending on levels of pain. Full weight bearing is allowed after 1 month. Postoperative dressing is minimized with fast healing (**Fig. 14**).

Results

Healing is achieved in 2 months. An average translation of 38% has been measured. The power of the translation was increased by 20% by the rotation of the posterior fragment. No neurologic or vascular lesion has been reported.

Discussion

Medial or lateral heel osteotomy is a common procedure. The usual procedure can be complicated with skin problems. To minimize risk, we have used a percutaneous approach for several years, which has proved to be an easy and reproducible procedure. To confirm this finding, we evaluated the reproducibility of the procedure with

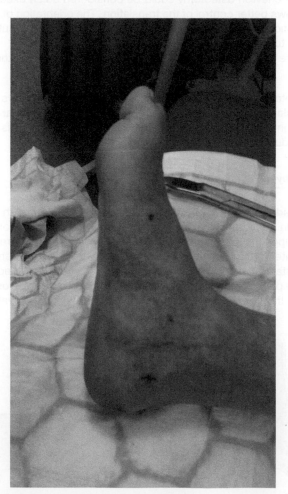

Fig. 14. The approach for percutaneous heel osteotomy.

1 day's training for surgeons. The results systematically showed complete osteotomy. The facility of the cut, the power of the translation, and the mobility of the osteotomy have been emphasized by the surgeons. Shifting the heel can be difficult, and some investigators have used a lamina spreader to free and mobilize the osteotomy. Because we use a 3-mm-wide burr, the spontaneous mobility of the osteotomy is impressive. Translation was easily obtained, with an average translation of 38%. With an average of 35 mm width, 38% resulted in a translation of 13 mm. The lever arm of a K-wire or a small periosteal elevator gives strength to translate the heel, but it also causes rotation, reported to average 20°. If the apex of the chevron is 15 mm posterior, a rotation of 20° means an additional translation of 5 mm. The translation obtained percutaneously is the equal at 18 mm.

Protection of the soft tissue with the Halsted, when the burr is introduced, is useful for preventing nerve damage. Because the burr is not longer than 20 mm, it can be completely introduced into the bone, leaving the noncutting part outside. In this condition, the only risk is using a high-speed burr and burning the soft tissue around the portal. The dissection showed no damage to the nerve.

Percutaneous chevron osteotomy could be considered as an excessive labor, but the V shape allows better control of the translation. The orientation of the apex determines the elevation, shortening, or lowering of the heel. A straight cut cannot control elevation of the tuberosity.

This procedure is quick and allows the operator to concentrate on the second stage.

Summary

Calcaneal osteotomy is a common procedure but the literature shows local complications such as skin necrosis, infection, and nerve lesion. A percutaneous approach avoids these complications with good reproducibility. Translation is as effective as the open procedure.

Zadek Osteotomy

Introduction

Pioneered by Zadek in 1939, this osteotomy is designed to control the position of the high tuberosity in a sagittal plane. It is a dorsal closing wedge osteotomy. It allows the posterior and superior angle of the tuberosity to be brought forward, reducing the conflict with the anterior face of the Achilles tendon. The position of the vertex of the wedge is important. It determines whether or not the heel is placed horizontally. If the vertex is kept posterior, a forward rotation of the high tuberosity is obtained (**Fig. 15**), but if the vertex is more anterior in the rotation, an elevation of the high

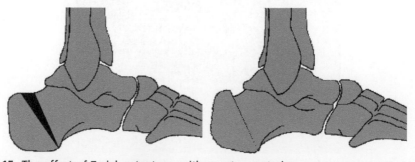

Fig. 15. The effect of Zadek osteotomy with a vertex posterior.

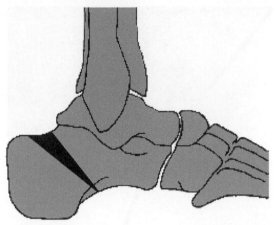

Fig. 16. Zadek osteotomy with a vertex anterior.

tuberosity is achieved (**Fig. 16**). The result is horizontalization of the heel (**Fig. 17**), particularly in cavus foot.

Technique

The procedure is performed with the patient lying in a lateral position (see **Fig. 1**). The operative foot is on top and is placed over the end of the table. The C-arm is positioned underneath (see **Fig. 3**). A thigh tourniquet is positioned. A popliteal block, spinal or general anesthesia is necessary.

The technique requires a Shannon burr 3 mm wide and 20 mm long, a wedge burr 3.1 mm wide and 12 mm long, a specific burr driver with high torque and low speed, and a pencil driver (see **Fig. 4**).

The wedge is planned preoperatively. To obtain a perfect osteotomy with the perfect degree, 2 K-wires are introduced percutaneously under fluoroscopic control and a dorsal wedge is defined. The vertex is carefully positioned (**Fig. 18**).

A short skin incision (6–7 mm) is made on the lateral side of the calcaneus in the middle of the wedge. The soft tissue is dissected with a Halsted until contact is made with

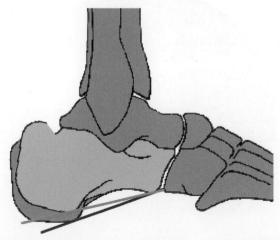

Fig. 17. The effect of the Zadek osteotomy with a vertex anterior: horizontalization of the heel. Blue line the position before the osteotomy. Green line the position after the osteotomy.

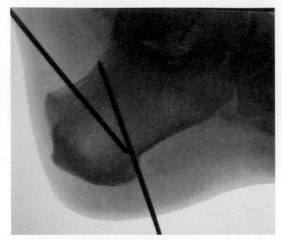

Fig. 18. The position of the 2 K-wires to obtain perfect osteotomy.

the bone. The clip is kept open to prevent nerve lesion until the burr is totally introduced in to the bone (see **Fig. 7**).

The osteotomy is performed at the speed of 350 rpm. Because of the width of the os calcis and the length of the burr, the osteotomy cannot be completed in 1 swipe. The bone is reamed until the burr is in contact with the posterior K-wire, and a straight cut is made on the lateral side and then on the medial side.

The anterior part of the wedge is then slowly reamed and progressively closed with the Shannon or the wedge. When the wedge is achieved, the K-wires are removed. The wedge is closed by dorsal flexion of the ankle. The osteotomy is fixed with 1 screw (**Fig. 19**).

The wound is closed with an absorbable suture.

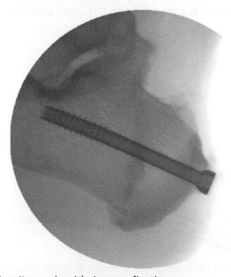

Fig. 19. The final radiograph with 1 screw fixation.

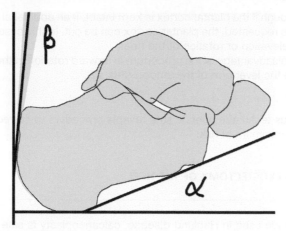

Fig. 20. Chauveaux and Liet (CL) measurement for Haglund deformity: CL=α–β.

Postoperative care

The foot is immobilized with a walking boot for 2 months. Partial weight bearing with crutches is permitted depending on levels of pain. Full weight bearing is allowed after 1 month. Postoperative dressing is minimized with fast healing.

Results

Healing is achieved in 2 months. The correction is stackable to the preoperative plane. No neurologic or vascular lesion has been reported.

Discussion

Designed to treat Haglund disease by forward rotation of the high tuberosity of the os calcis, Zadek osteotomy is not frequently performed, as shown by the lack of publications. More common in France, it is an alternative to a simple exostectomy. Many algorithms have been used to define one procedure or another according to different measurements. With the algorithm of Chauveaux and Liet,[1] an angle superior to 30° is a good indication for a primary Zadek osteotomy (**Fig. 20**). The procedure is often used as a secondary procedure after failure of a simple exostectomy. Its attraction is the potential to horizontalize the heel by displacing the vertex anteriorly. Each degree of the wedge elevates the posterior tuberosity by the same degree (**Fig. 21**).

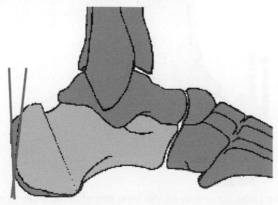

Fig. 21. Effect of the Zadek, dorsal closing wedge, on the posterior tuberosity: rotation of the tuberosity.

One screw is enough if the plantar cortex is kept intact. If an additional elevation of the high tuberosity is requested, the plantar cortex can be cut. In this case, 2 screws prevent excessive elevation or rotation of the heel.

The potential disadvantage of the procedure is forward rotation of the Achilles insertion to decrease the lever arm of the tendon (**Fig. 22**).

Summary
The percutaneous technique offers a safe reliable procedure to correct the deformity precisely with a minimum of risk.

PERCUTANEOUS EXOSTECTOMY OF THE HEEL
Calcaneoplasty

Introduction
The main technique used in Haglund disease, calcaneoplasty is safe and easy. Performed initially with an open lateral approach, different procedures have been described, such as arthroscopy and a percutaneous approach. Endoscopic calcaneoplasty was described by van Dijk in 2001[2] and quickly spread throughout Europe and worldwide. Using a double posterior approach in a prone position, it offers a permanent control of the view and a less aggressive dissection. For 20 years, Mariano de Prado, Stephen Isham, and more recently, GRECMIP (Groupe de Recherche et d'Etude en Chirurgie Mini-Invasive du Pied [Group of Research and Study in Minimally Invasive Surgery of the Foot]) have offered training in percutaneous calcaneoplasty.

Technique
The procedure is performed with the patient lying in a lateral position (see **Fig. 1**). The operative foot is on top and is placed over the end of the table. The C-arm is positioned underneath (see **Fig. 3**). No tourniquet is necessary. A popliteal block, spinal or general anesthesia is necessary.

The technique requires a wedge burr 3.1 mm wide and 12 mm long, a specific burr driver with high torque and low speed, and a pencil driver (see **Fig. 4**).

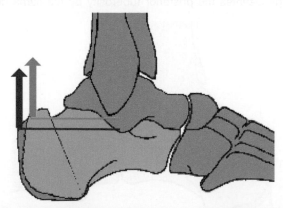

Fig. 22. Effect of the Zadek osteotomy on the lever arm of the Achilles tendon. The blue line and arrow reflect the action of the tendon before the osteotomy and the green line and arrow, its action after the osteotomy.

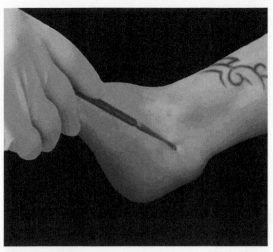

Fig. 23. Calcaneoplasty, the percutaneous approach.

The incision is made, with a Beaver blade, lateral to the Achilles tendon and distal at the level of the insertion (**Fig. 23**). The position is controlled with a fluoroscope.

A small periosteal elevator is introduced through the incision to create an appropriate working area against the tuberosity.

With fluoroscopic control, the wedge is gently introduced against the bone (**Fig. 24**). At a low speed, the protuberance is shaved. Because of the level of the incision, the instruments are introduced oblique plantar to dorsal. When the calcaneoplasty is complete, the burr will end up vertical.

Shaving or reaming the bone creates debris and paste, which must be removed (**Fig. 25**). A small specific rasp is inserted, and progressively, the cavity is cleaned of all the pieces of bone. A cannula is then positioned against the bone at the bottom

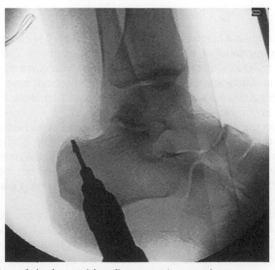

Fig. 24. Introduction of the burr with a fluoroscopic control.

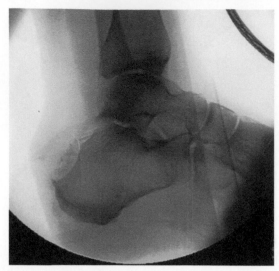

Fig. 25. Bone debris must be cleaned.

of the work space and saline is flushed copiously from inside to outside, taking away the remaining pieces.

Fluoroscopic control is helpful to verify the quality of the resection.

Postoperative care

The foot is immobilized with a walking boot for 1 month. Full weight bearing with crutches is allowed immediately depending on levels of pain. Postoperative dressing is minimized with fast healing.

Results

No neurologic or vascular lesion has been reported. The results are similar to the open technique.

Discussion

The Haglund deformity is a common condition in foot and ankle clinics. Its treatment is reliable in different procedures, such as simple exostectomy or Zadek osteotomy. A simple exostectomy allows quick and simple recovery, because the structure of the foot is not changed. Many approaches haves been described: open lateral, posterior trans-Achilles, arthroscopic, or percutaneous. The last two allow limited dissection and less cutaneous complication.

Although the percutaneous procedure seems to be quick and easy, it is necessary to be meticulous during both shaving and cleaning. While the posterior tuberosity is being reamed, a regular sweeping movement avoids digging the os calcis too deeply. If the shape of the burr is made to aggress only the bone and not the tissue, you can damage the insertion of the achilles tendon. Fluoroscopic controls are essential to prevent this problem.

Paste and debris of bone are the source of inflammatory response and secondary ossification. They must be conscientiously removed. Large pieces of bone can be extracted with a clip and the smaller ones taken away with a specific rasp. Adequate washing is essential; a large amount of fluid is necessary to clear the working space.

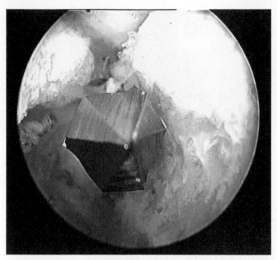

Fig. 26. Mixed procedure: arthroscopy and percutaneous.

Two points can be discussed — the percutaneous procedure could be blamed as being responsible for a possible inflammatory reaction because the bursitis is not excised. Secondly, at any time the Achilles tendon is not perfectly controlled. To avoid these problems, a mixed arthroscopy and percutaneous procedure can be adopted (**Fig. 26**). First, endoscopy allows complete excision of the bursitis and identification of an insertional tendinopathy. The working area is created with a shaver. Then, calcaneoplasty is quickly performed percutaneously. The exostectomy is controlled arthroscopically and the cavity is cleaned. The procedure is performed supine with a medial and a lateral approach more distal than those described by van Dijk.[2] Because the procedure includes arthroscopy, it is controlled under the view and the fluoroscopic time is reduced. With increasing experience, its use becomes unnecessary.

Summary
Percutaneous calcaneoplasty offers a quick (15 minutes) and reliable procedure, although fluoroscopic control is needed. Mixing arthroscopy and percutaneous procedures offers the reliability of both, the quick operating time of the percutaneous approach, and the view control and lack of radiation of arthroscopy.

Plantar Fasciitis Exostectomy

Introduction
Usually treated with medical recommendations such as stretching, physiotherapy, and cortisone injections, plantar fasciitis can be resistant to treatment. Different surgical techniques have been described as open or arthroscopic sections. A percutaneous procedure involving the shaving of the spur can be used.

Technique
The procedure is performed with the patient lying in a lateral position (see **Fig. 1**). The operative foot is on top and is placed over the end of the table. The C-arm is positioned underneath (see **Fig. 3**). No tourniquet is necessary. A popliteal block or spinal or general anesthesia is needed.

The technique requires a wedge burr 3.1 mm wide and 12 mm long, a specific burr driver with high torque and low speed, and a pencil driver (see **Fig. 4**).

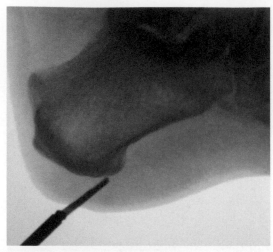

Fig. 27. Position of the approach for plantar fasciitis.

The incision follows a line parallel to the plantar side of the calcaneus to the bottom and the middle of the heel. At the beginning of the learning curve, it is helpful to use a fluoroscope (**Fig. 27**).

The wedge burr is introduced against the bone to shave the calcaneus spur.

Shaving or reaming the bone creates debris and paste, which must be removed. A small specific rasp is inserted, and progressively, the cavity is cleaned of all pieces of bone. A cannula is then positioned against the bone at the bottom of the work space and saline is flushed copiously from inside to outside, taking away the remaining pieces.

Postoperative care
A simple dressing is needed. Full weight bearing with crutches is immediately permitted depending on the levels of pain.

Discussion
A simple and quick procedure, exostectomy has a double action: section of the plantar fascia and removal of the spur. If excision of the bone is not a priority, the psychological effect on the patient is real.

Summary
Percutaneous techniques have been reported since they were introduced by Poliakov in 1945. They have evolved in parallel with open surgery and biotechnology, specific burrs and drills, and powerful screws. Combining these techniques with classic fixed osteotomy presents many more possibilities for correction, with the advantages of a quick, less invasive and more reliable procedure, offering the patient improved adaptability. These techniques represent another useful tool in the box of the foot and ankle surgeon.

REFERENCES

1. Chauveaux D, Liet P, Le Huec JC, et al. A new radiologic measurement for the diagnosis of Haglund's deformity. Surg Radiol Anat 1991;13:39–44.
2. Van Dijk CN, Scholten PE, Krips R. A 2-portal endoscopic approach for diagnosis and treatment of posterior ankle pathology. Technical note. Arthroscopy 2000;16: 871–6.

Supramalleolar Osteotomies

An Algorithm for the Deformed Ankle

Melissa M. Galli, DPM, MHA, AACFAS[a], Ryan T. Scott, DPM, FACFAS[b],*

KEYWORDS

- Tibial osteotomy • Fibular osteotomy • Congenital deformity
- Posttraumatic deformity • Ankle arthritis

KEY POINTS

- Understand the importance of appropriate preoperative planning for supramalleolar osteotomies.
- Surgical procedures and fixation techniques for correction of a varus/valgus ankle joint.
- Differentiate between the pros and cons of a fibular versus tibial osteotomy.

INTRODUCTION: NATURE OF THE PROBLEM

Supramalleolar osteotomies (SMO) are powerful osteotomies that realign the tibiotalar and optimize hindfoot position in the presence of varus, valgus, procurvatum, recurvatum, as well as internal and external rotation of the tibia. Although used in the pediatric and hemophilic population earlier, SMO is a relatively new reconstructive surgical technique that was introduced by Takakura and colleagues[1] in 1995. Conducted primarily in cancellous bone, SMOs offer rapid, reliable bony consolidation compared with dome osteotomies and complex arthrodesis.

Although high tibial osteotomies of the tibial plateau have been described to treat symptomatic ankle deformity when the mechanical axis passes through an asymptomatic knee, for the simplicity of this SMO discussion, only osteotomies distal to the mid-diaphysis of the tibia and fibula are addressed.[2] Ultimately, a consensus on the acceptable limits of angular deformity of the tibia and the potential development of a symptomatic, arthritic ankle joint do not exist[3–5]; as such, symptomatic or a nonbraceable asymptomatic asymmetric deformity is a mandatory requirement for all SMO indications, in the authors' opinion.

Complex foot and ankle deformity is typically caused by congenital (clubfoot, vertical talus), neurologic (poliomyelitis, cerebral palsy, meningomyelocele), traumatic

[a] Department of Orthopedics, The CORE Institute, 18444 North 25th Avenue, Suite 210, Phoenix, AZ 85023-1264, USA; [b] Department of Orthopedics, The CORE Institute, 18444 North 25th Avenue, Suite 320, Phoenix, AZ 85023, USA
* Corresponding author.
E-mail address: scottryt@gmail.com

Clin Podiatr Med Surg 32 (2015) 435–444
http://dx.doi.org/10.1016/j.cpm.2015.03.005   podiatric.theclinics.com
0891-8422/15/$ – see front matter © 2015 Elsevier Inc. All rights reserved.

pathologic conditions, osteomyelitis, nonunion or malunion, leg length discrepancy, burn contractures, and other soft tissue contractures.[6–15] Tibial malalignment results in awkward gait, excessive shoe wear, and difficulties in orthoses. Furthermore, it has been shown in biomechanical studies to decrease the contact area of the tibiotalar joint up to 40%[3] and to affect tibiotalar contact shape and contact location.[16] In the younger patient, the effects of abnormal tibial torsion may be cosmetic and functional. Most patients present with excessive in-toeing or out-toeing and may also complain of tripping, leg pain, poor endurance, or brace intolerance.[17] In the pediatric population, conventional treatment of these deformities includes soft tissue releases, tendon transfers, osteotomies, and arthrodesis.[6,9,11–15]

After physeal closure, the indications for SMO are peri-articular deformities of the distal tibia, malunited ankle arthrodesis, and talar or subtalar deformities with concomitant ankle arthrosis[6,7,9,11–15] or asymptomatic ankle osteoarthritis with concomitant valgus or varus deformity and a partially (at least 50%) preserved tibiotalar joint surface.[18–20] With all SMOs used in arthritic indications, the thought process is to redistribute weight-bearing forces to a healthier aspect of the cartilage. Thus, SMOs are ideal to re-establish the mechanical axis of the ankle and minimize the progression of ankle arthritis when reasonable preoperative ankle range of motion is present.[21]

In older patients, the SMO has several advantages. It avoids neurovascular complications seen in roughly 29% of all proximal tibial osteotomies[18,22] and allows the simultaneous correction of ankle varus/valgus by the removal of the appropriate bony wedge.[18,23,24] Historically, opening/closing wedge osteotomies of the medial and lateral tibia are the most used osteotomies in multiplanar correction.[25] The medial and lateral approach is based on the amount of correction desired.[26] The medial opening wedge osteotomy has the advantages of using a simple approach, ease of bone cuts, and no resultant limb length discrepancy. The lateral closing wedge osteotomy allows for ease of fixation, no graft requirement, reliable and rapid healing, and no possibility of medial joint load increase.[27] Recently, a multiplanar dome-shaped osteotomy has been described in the correction in the varus or valgus ankle.[28]

The location, type, and size of osteotomy required are based on the angular deformity and the center of rotation and angulation (CORA). Each osteotomy has to be carefully planned out, including fixation options (screws, plates, staples) (**Figs. 1** and **2**). Internal fixation[29] for the management of the SMO may be ill-suited for larger or more complex deformity correction, whereas the use of external fixation allows for a gradual correction over time and prevents acute stretching of the neurovascular structures or the creation of large opening-wedge gaps requiring bone grafting.[6,11–13]

The need for fibular SMO in conjunction with tibial SMO remains controversial for some deformities, yet in some, like ankle valgus, without it correction would be difficult if not impossible to maintain. According to Inan and colleagues,[30] "theoretically, excessive derotation of the distal tibia in the presence of an intact fibula can lead to incongruity of the ankle" (**Table 1**).

The absolute contraindication for an isolated SMO realignment surgery is end-stage degenerative changes of the complete tibiotalar joint, unmanageable hindfoot instability, acute or chronic infections, severe vascular or neurologic deficiency, and neuropathic disorders.[18] Other contraindications include a talar tilt 7.3° to 10° or greater.[13,37] In these scenarios, the SMO has not been found to be as effective for correction.[38]

SURGICAL TECHNIQUE

Preoperative planning is imperative to obtaining optimal results and, often, takes more time than the procedure itself. Standing long leg films, dedicated weight bearing (WB)

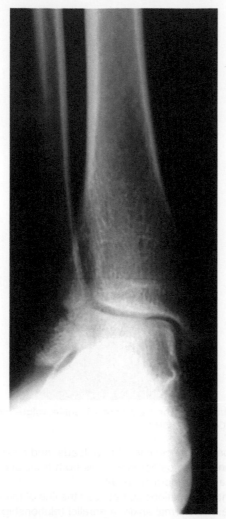

Fig. 1. Postoperative tibial SMO for treatment of ankle valgus deformity. (*Courtesy of* C. Hyer, DPM, FACFAS, Columbus, OH.)

ankle films, Saltzman views, WB lateral, and anteroposterior (AP) of the foot are ordered to ensure apex of the deformity is identified.[39–41] In addition, AP, medial oblique (MO), and lateral WB ankle films of the contralateral ankle are ordered to determine optimal fibular length and rotation. In the normal ankle, the tip of the lateral malleolus is 3 to 4 mm lower than that of the medial malleolus; the Shenton line is intact, and the "dime sign" is present at the lateral malleolar tip.[31,42]

The standard ankle angles should be analyzed on a standing AP of the ankle:

- CORA is the intersection of the mechanical axis of the proximal and distal segments making up deformity.[43] If possible, closing or opening wedge should be planned at the level of CORA to allow complete alignment of the foot and ankle. If the osteotomy must be made proximal or distal to CORA, the center of the tibiotalar joint will translate relative to the mechanical axis of the tibia. In this

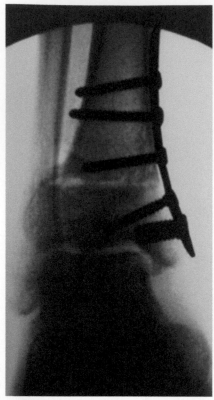

Fig. 2. Preoperative tibial SMO for treatment of ankle valgus deformity. (*Courtesy of* C. Hyer, DPM, FACFAS, Columbus, OH.)

case, there will be an unnecessary shift of loads, and a clinical zigzag deformity will be created unless the osteotomy line is both translated and angulated.

- Lateral distal tibial angle (normal 86–92°)
- Talar tilt represents the relationship between the line of the tibial plafond and that of the talar dome. In a normal ankle, a parallel relationship exists.[31]

Table 1
Fibular supramalleolar osteotomy pros and cons

Fibular SMO Pros	Fibular SMO Cons
The distal fibula is known to play a pivotal role in anatomic reduction of the ankle joint, helps restore ankle stability and congruity of the mortise[31–33]	Incidence of malunion after fibular reconstruction is up to 33%[34]
In cases of open epiphyses, an isolated tibial SMO may cause recurrence of the rotational deformity. Thus, fibular SMO is oft advocated in this population	Banks and Evans[35] and Ryan and colleagues[36] have described full tibial SMO derotation techniques without utilization of fibular SMO so may not be necessary
—	An intact fibula has been shown to provide additional support of the osteotomized tibia and, particularly, protects against sagittal plane angulation[35,36]

The need for fibular SMO is diagnosed based on comparative contralateral ankle films:

- Talocrural angle captures the tibial plafond and the line through the tips of the malleoli. If the difference of this angle is 3° or greater between the affected and contralateral extremity, fibular shortening is present.[31]
- The bimalleolar angle is a relationship connecting the malleolar tips and a vertical line following the fibular intra-medullary space, immediately superior to the ankle joint. A difference of 2.5° or greater between sides suggests fibular shortening.[31]

MRI is only required when analyzing soft tissue and articular cartilage, and single-photon emission computed tomography-computed tomography (SPECT-CT) can be used to determine areas of increased tibiotalar joint pressure. Bilateral CT scan is used to measure the length of the tibia and fibula accurately:

- Tibiofibular length ratio can be calculated.[42]
- Accurate fibular placement of the lateral malleolus in the incisura fibularis tibiae can be confirmed or malrotation identified (**Fig. 3**).[31]

PREPARATION AND PATIENT POSITIONING

The procedure is performed under general anesthesia with or without a regional block for postoperative pain control.[44] The patient is placed supine with a thigh tourniquet with or without hip rotation based on concomitant procedures. For isolated tibial SMO, the authors recommend the tibial tuberosity face due north on the operating room table. Given the nature of the deformity and the need for wide-angled intraoperative radiographs, the authors recommend using a large C-arm versus a mini C-arm.

SURGICAL APPROACH AND PROCEDURE

1. If SMO at CORA, make an incision directly over the predetermined site preoperatively approximately 4 to 6 cm in length.[45] To preserve enough bone for placement of the plate, the osteotomy should always be placed at least 2.5 cm above the tibiotalar joint. If SMO is not at CORA, medial osteotomy is 4 to 5 cm proximal to the medial malleolar tip and the incision lies directly overhead.
2. Minimal periosteal stripping should be performed on all incisions. Two 2-mm Kirschner (K)-wires are inserted as osteotomy guides and confirmed radiographically.
3. An opening wedge, horizontal cut to the tibia via a broad oscillating saw should be performed under fluoroscopy. Carefully preserve the opposite cortex and periosteal sleeve to act as a fulcrum for the opening wedge and to enhance stability if performed at CORA. If not, the opposite cortex will need to be broken to allow for translation. A lamina spreader should be used to open the osteotomy until correction is achieved and confirmed radiographically. An appropriately shaped graft is then applied and fixated, most often via staples or buttress plating. If a wedge plate is used, the osteotomy site is backfilled with cancellous bone allograft.
4. A closing wedge and K-wires should be inserted as preosteotomy planning. The first K-wire is inserted perpendicular to the mechanical axis, and the second is inserted parallel to the ankle joint line intersecting the first wire at the apex of the deformity. The position should be confirmed radiographically and used as guides for tibial cuts via an oscillating saw. All osteotomies must be fixed with periarticular plating or staples.

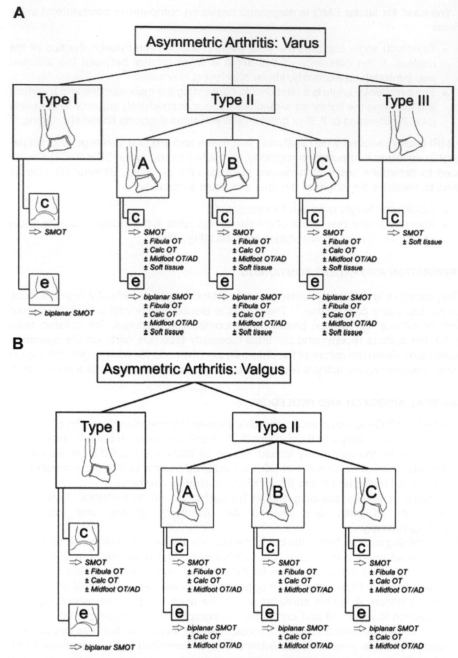

Fig. 3. (A and B) Classification and treatment algorithm for SMOs. AD, arthrodesis; OT, osteotomy; SMOT, supramalleolar osteotomy. (*Adapted from* Knupp M, Stufkens SA, Bollinger L, et al. Classification of treatment of supramalleolar deformities. Foot Ankle Int 2011:32(11);1024–5; with permission.)

5. If needed, fibular osteotomy should be performed at the level of the tibial osteotomy (before or after tibial based on deformity). Oblique osteotomy is created through a small 5-cm lateral longitudinal incision with protection of the syndesmosis. Next, 2.5-mm K-wires are placed from an anterolateral direction with approximately 60° to the coronal plane in the proximal and distal fibula to the osteotomy for segmental distraction via a distractor. Appropriate radiographic positioning of the fibula is confirmed radiographically by the following criteria:
   a. Appropriate closure of the medial clear space with restoration of the relationship of the medial malleolus and the medial surface of the talus
   b. An anatomic position of the talus within the mortise with parallel articular surfaces of the tibiotalar joint
   c. Restoration of the anatomic landmarks as stated by Weber and Simpson[46]
6. After realignment of the tibiotalar axis, one must fully assess the hindfoot and over-all foot position via simulated weight-bearing intraoperative radiographs. Associated inframalleolar osteotomies and adjunctive soft tissue balancing procedures may be required, especially in the incongruent ankle.[47]

IMMEDIATE POSTOPERATIVE CARE

Isolated closing SMO fixed with a staple postoperative care is a well-padded below-knee walking cast with 48 hours of bed rest, followed by 2 weeks of partially weight-bearing and then full weight-bearing for 4 weeks.[48] The cast is removed at 6 weeks. In cases of opening SMO requiring graft incorporation, patients are kept non-weight-bearing or partially weight-bearing until there is evidence of radiographic healing. In SMO with distraction arthoplasty, the foot ring is removed at 12 weeks at the end of the distraction period and the remainder of fixator is removed when adequate healing is obtained of the SMO (mean 16 weeks with range from 12 to 18).[49]

Although most investigators recommend plain film radiographs for evaluation of SMO healing, some[20] recommend SPECT-CT scans at 6 months to assess union after primary surgery.

REHABILITATION AND RECOVERY

Early range of motion without resistance and non-weight-bearing strengthening of the extremity proximal to the surgical site is initiated in all cases without preclusion of concomitant procedures. Once osseous healing is confirmed, resistance is added to ranging exercises, and WB strengthening of the extremity with exercises crossing the ankle joint is instituted.[3]

CLINICAL RESULTS IN THE LITERATURE

Most of the literature supports osteotomies of the tibia for management of deformity of the ankle. Concomitant literature is also present on the importance of the lateral malleolus in normal ankle anatomy.[27,50] Correction of supramalleolar malalignment helps normalize the intra-articular load distribution and thereby diminish excessive asymmetric cartilage load.[51] By manipulating the distal fibula into a varus or valgus position by 1°, the contact area of the tibiotalar joint is reduced by more than 50% showing the importance of the fibula in SMO.[52] Knupp and colleagues[53] evaluated the intra-articular pressures with varying SMOs. They note the importance of the medial and lateral collateral ligaments in stabilizing the varus and valgus ankle. They also conclude that isolated distal tibial realignment maybe the main step in normalizing the force pressure within the ankle joint. Recognition of hindfoot malalignment is pivotal because 63% of the patients with ankle joint arthritis present with a malaligned hindfoot.[51,54] Clinical studies examining SMO in patient populations encompassing cerebral palsy, spina bifida, heomophilic, postpronational external rotation ankle fracture malunions, and varus and valgus ankle deformities are prolific throughout the literature with short- to midterm follow-up. SMO's have been found to reduce pain, preserve tibiotalar function, increased American Orthopaedic Foot and Ankle Society scores by an average of 25 points from before operation to after operation with minimal deformity reoccurrence.[3,45,48,55,56]

SUMMARY

SMO is indicated in isolation in cases of reasonable ankle function and even in the presence of mild arthritic changes. SMO with concomitant procedures broadens the corrective power and is indicated in cases of advanced degenerative joint pathologic abnormality. Regardless of the cause of the deformity, optimal results depend on anatomic restoration of the ankle mortise by adequate lengthening and correction of rotational and angular deformity as well as an optimal hindfoot position and functionality.[6,7,9–12,45]

REFERENCES

1. Takakura Y, Tanaka Y, Kumai T, et al. Low tibial osteotomy for osteoarthritis of the ankle. Results of a new operation in 18 patients. J Bone Joint Surg Br 1995;77(1): 50–4.
2. Elson DW, Paweleck JE, Shields DW, et al. Stretching the indications: high tibial osteotomy used successfully to treat isolated ankle symptoms. BMJ Case Rep 2013;2013 [pii:bcr2013200527].
3. Stamatis ED, Cooper PS, Myerson MS. Supramalleolar osteotomy for the treatment of distal tibial angular deformities and arthritis of the ankle joint. Foot Ankle Int 2003;24(10):754–64.
4. Kristensen KD, Kiaer T, Blicher J. No arthrosis of the ankle 20 years after malaligned tibial-shaft fracture. Acta Orthop Scand 1989;60:208–9.
5. Merchant TC, Dietz FR. Long-term follow-up after fractures of the tibial and fibular shafts. J Bone Joint Surg Am 1989;71:599–606.
6. Sen C, Kocaoglu M, Eralp L, et al. Correction of ankle and hindfoot deformities by supramalleolar osteotomy. Foot Ankle Int 2003;24(1):22–8.
7. Calhoun JH, Evans EB, Herndon DN. Techniques for the management of burn contractures with the Ilizarov Fixator. Clin Orthop 1992;280:117–24.
8. Grant AD, Atar D, Lehman WB. The Ilizarov technique in correction of complex foot deformities. Clin Orthop 1992;280:94–103.
9. Herzenberg JE, Smith JD, Paley D. Correcting torsional deformities with Ilizarov's apparatus. Clin Orthop Relat Res 1994;302:36–41.
10. Kocaoglu M, Eralp L, Atalar AC, et al. The treatment of complex foot deformities by the Ilizarov method. Acta Orthop Traumatol Turc 2001;35(1):63–70.
11. Paley D. The correction of complex foot deformities using Ilizarov's distraction osteotomies. Clin Orthop 1993;293:97–111.
12. Paley D. Priniciples of complex foot deformities correction: Ilizarov technique. In: Gould JS, editor. Operative foot surgery. Philadelphia: WB Saunders; 1994. p. 476–514.
13. Paley D, Herzenberg JE. Applications of external fixation to foot and ankle reconstruction. In: Myerson M, editor. Foot principles of deformity correction. 1st edition. New York: Springer-Verlag; 2002. p. 571–635.

14. Paley D. Ankle malalignment. In: Kelikian A, editor. Operative treatment of the foot and ankle. Stanford (CA): Appleton and lange; 1999. p. 547–86.
15. Paley D. Ankle and foot considerations. In: Paley D, editor. Principles of deformity correction. 1st edition. New York: Springer-Verlag; 2002. p. 571–642.
16. Tarr RR, Resnick CT, Wagner KS, et al. Changes in tibiotalar joint contract areas following experimentally induced tibial angular deformities. Clin Orthop 1985;199: 72–80.
17. Selber P, Filho ER, Dallalana R, et al. Supramalleolar derotation osteotomy of the tibia, with T plate fixation. J Bone Joint Surg Br 2004;86(8):1170–5.
18. Barg A, Pagenstert GI, Horisberger M, et al. Supramalleolar osteotomies for degenerative joint disease of the ankle joint: indication, technique, and results. Int Orthop 2013;37:1683–95.
19. Easley ME. Surgical treatment of the arthritic varus ankle. Foot Ankle Clin 2012; 17(4):665–86.
20. Barg A, Pagenstert GI, Leumann AG, et al. Treatment of the arthritic valgus ankle. Foot Ankle Clin 2012;17(4):647–63.
21. Weatherall JM, Mroczek K, McLaurin T, et al. Post-traumatic ankle arthritis. Bull Hosp Jt Dis 2013;71(1):104–12.
22. Steel HH, Sandrow RE, Sullivan PD. Complications of tibial osteotomy in children with genu varum or valgum: evidence that neurological changes are due to ischemia. J Bone Joint Surg Am 1971;53:1629–35.
23. Fraser RK, Menelaus MB. The management of tibial torsion in patients with spina bifida. J Bone Joint Surg Br 1993;75:495–7.
24. Krengel WF 3rd, Staheli LT. Tibial rotational osteotomy for idiopathic torsion: a comparison of the proximal and distal osteotomy levels. Clin Orthop 1992;283:285–9.
25. Nelman K, Weiner DS, Morcher MA, et al. Multiplanar supramalleolar osteotomy in the management of complex rigid foot deformities in children. J Child Orthop 2009;3:39–46.
26. Knupp M, Stufkens SA, Bollinger L, et al. Classification of treatment of supramalleolar deformities. Foot Ankle Int 2011;32(11):1023–31.
27. Harstall R, Lehman O, Krause F, et al. Supramalleolar lateral closing wedge osteotomy for the treatment of varus ankle arthrosis. Foot Ankle Int 2007;28(5): 542–8.
28. Colin F, Wagner P, Bollinger L, et al. Tibia dome-shaped osteotomy for a valgus deformity in a ball-and-socket ankle joint: a case report. Clin Res Foot Ankle 2013;1(2):1–3.
29. McNicol D, Leong JC, Hsu LC. Supramalleolar derotation osteotomy for lateral tibial torsion and associated equinovarus deformity of the foot. J Bone Joint Surg Br 1983;65(2):166–70.
30. Inan M, Ferri-de Baros F, Chan G, et al. Correction of rotational deformity of the tibia in cerebral palsy by percutaneous supramalleolar osteotomy. J Bone Joint Surg Br 2005;87(10):1411–5.
31. van Wensen RJ, van den Bekerom MP, Marti RK, et al. Reconstructive osteotomy of fibular malunion: review of the literature. Strategies Traum Limb Reconstr 2011; 6:51–7.
32. Yablon IG, Heller FG, Shouse L. The key role of the lateral malleolus in displaced fractures of the ankle. J Bone Joint Surg Am 1977;59(2):169–73.
33. Marti RK, Raaymakers EL, Nolte PA. Malunited ankle fractures. The late results of reconstruction. J Bone Joint Surg Br 1990;72(4):709–13.
34. Chu A, Weiner L. Distal fibula malunions. J Am Acad Orthop Surg 2009;17(4): 220–30.

35. Banks SW, Evans EA. Simple transverse osteotomy and threaded-pin fixation for controlled correction of torsion deformities of the tibia. J Bone Joint Surg Am 1955;37:193–5.
36. Ryan DD, Rethlefsen SA, Skaggs DL, et al. Results of tibial rotational osteotomy without concomitant fibular osteotomy in children with cerebral palsy. J Pediatr Orthop 2005;25:84–8.
37. Frigg A, Jud L, Valderrabano V. Intraoperative positioning of the hindfoot with the hindfoot alignment guide: a pilot study. Foot Ankle Int 2014;35(1):56–62.
38. Lee WC, Ahn JY, Cho JH, et al. Realignment surgery for severe talar tilt secondary to paralytic cavovarus. Foot Ankle Int 2013;34(11):1552–9.
39. Stevens PM, Kennedy JM, Hung M. Guided growth for ankle valgus. J Pediatr Orthop 2011;31(8):878–83.
40. Stevens PM. Effect of ankle valgus on radiographic appearance of the ankle. J Pediatr Orthop 1988;8:184–6.
41. Machen MS, Stevens PM. Should full-length standing anteroposterior radiographs replace the scanogram for measurement of limb length discrepancy? J Pediatr Orthop 2005;14:30–7.
42. Malhotra D, Puri R, Owen R. Valgus deformity of the ankle in children with spina bifida aperta. J Bone Joint Surg Br 1984;66(3):381–5.
43. Ellington JK, Myerson MS. Surgical correction of the ball and socket ankle joint in the adult associated with a talonavicular tarsal coalition. Foot Ankle Int 2013; 34(10):1381–8.
44. Valderrabano V, Paul J, Monika H, et al. Joint-preserving surgery of valgus ankle osteoarthritis. Foot Ankle Clin N Am 2013;18:481–502.
45. Hintermann B, Barg A, Knupp M. Corrective supramalleolar osteotomy for malunited pronation-external rotation fractures of the ankle. J Bone Joint Surg Br 2011;93(10):1367–72.
46. Weber BG, Simpson LA. Corrective lengthening osteotomy of the fibula. Clin Orthop 1985;199:61–7.
47. Trincat S, Kouyoumdjian P, Asencio G. Total ankle arthroplasty and coronal plane deformities. Ortho Traumatol Surg Res 2012;98:75–84.
48. Pearce MS, Smith MA, Savidge GF. Supramalleolar tibial osteotomy for haemophilic arthropathy of the ankle. J Bone Joint Surg Br 1994;76(6):947–50.
49. Tellisi N, Fragomen AT, Kleinman D, et al. Joint preservation of the osteoarthritic ankle using distraction arthroplasty. Foot Ankle Int 2009;30(4):318–25.
50. Kang SH, Rhee SK, Song SW, et al. Ankle deformity secondary to acquired fibular segmental defect in children. Clin Orthop Surg 2010;2:179–85.
51. Knupp M, Hintermann B. Treatment of asymmetric arthritis of the ankle joint with supramalleolar osteotomies. Foot Ankle Int 2012;33(3):250–2.
52. Stufkens SA, van Bergen CJ, Blankevoort L, et al. The role of the fibula in varus and valgus deformity of the tibia. J Bone Joint Surg Br 2011;93(9):1232–9.
53. Knupp M, Stufkens SA, van Bergen CJ, et al. Effect of supramalleolar varus and valgus deformities on the tibiotalar joint: a cadaveric study. Foot Ankle Int 2011; 32(6):609–15.
54. Valderrabano V, Hintermann B, Horisberger M, et al. Ligamentous posttraumatic ankle osteoarthritis. Am J Sports Med 2006;34(4):612–20.
55. Park JT, Eorn JS, Jung HG. Supramalleolar tibial osteotomy for medial compartment ankle osteoarthritis. J Korean Orthop Assoc 2013;48(2):89–95.
56. Horn DM, Fragomen AT, Rozbruch SR. Supramalleolar osteotomy using circular external fixation with six-axis deformity correction of the distal tibia. Foot Ankle Int 2011;32(10):986–93.

Supramalleolar Osteotomy
Indications and Surgical Techniques

Jennifer L. Mulhern, DPM[a], Nicole M. Protzman, MS[b], Stephen A. Brigido, DPM[a],*, Premjit Pete S. Deol, DO[c]

KEYWORDS

- Ankle arthritis • Asymmetric arthritis • Ankle realignment surgery
- Joint-preserving surgery • Supramalleolar osteotomy • Tibiotalar joint • Varus ankle

KEY POINTS

- Patients with ankle valgus or varus deformity have altered static and dynamic pressure distributions that can lead to asymmetric ankle osteoarthritis.
- Appropriate patient selection is paramount to the success of this procedure; the clinician must carefully consider the contraindications and any concomitant deformities or instabilities.
- Thorough preoperative planning is required to assess the origin of the deformity and calculate the extent of surgical correction.
- Research has confirmed the effectiveness of supramalleolar osteotomies to achieve anatomic correction with few complications and resultant improvements in pain and functionality.

INTRODUCTION

End-stage ankle joint arthritis is a painful and disabling condition that is most commonly precipitated by trauma.[1–3] Following exhaustion of conservative treatment, the surgeon must decide whether to perform a joint-sacrificing or joint-sparing procedure. With years of routine employment, ankle arthrodesis and total ankle replacement (TAR) have proved viable surgical alternatives. Even so, these joint-sacrificing procedures may not afford lifelong relief in younger patients. Therefore, in younger, more active patients, joint-sparing procedures may be a more optimal operative solution.

Disclosure Statement: Dr S.A. Brigido serves on the surgery advisory board for Alliqua and Bacterin International. He also serves as a consultant for Stryker. Alliqua, Bacterin International, and Stryker had no knowledge or influence in study design, protocol, or data collection.
ª Foot and Ankle Department, Coordinated Health, 2775 Schoenersville Road, Bethlehem, PA 18017, USA; ᵇ Clinical Education and Research Department, Coordinated Health, 3435 Winchester Road, Allentown, PA 18104, USA; ᶜ Orthopaedics Department, Panorama Orthopedics & Spine Center, 660 Golden Ridge Road, Suite 250, Golden, CO 80401, USA
* Corresponding author.
E-mail address: drsbrigido@mac.com

Clin Podiatr Med Surg 32 (2015) 445–461
http://dx.doi.org/10.1016/j.cpm.2015.03.006   podiatric.theclinics.com

Examples of joint-sparing procedures include arthroscopic debridement, arthrotomy, distraction arthroplasty, ligament reconstruction, resurfacing procedures, and corrective osteotomies.[4]

The supramalleolar osteotomy (SMO) of the tibia is a joint-sparing treatment option for the management of midstage, asymmetric arthritis of the ankle. The primary goal of the procedure is to re-establish the mechanical axis and anatomic relationships of the lower extremity to re-create a more even load distribution across the ankle.[5–11] In doing so, proper biomechanics are restored with resultant improvements in pain and function.[4–6,9–24] Herein, the present report discusses the key aspects of the SMO, including the surgical indications and contraindications, the principles of preoperative planning, the surgical techniques, and rehabilitation protocols; and lastly, the clinical results are reviewed.

Indications

Appropriate patient selection is paramount to successful outcomes. **Table 1** outlines the indications and contraindications for the procedure.[7,15,25–28]

SURGICAL TECHNIQUE
Preoperative Planning

SMOs are indicated for deformities located within the distal tibia and at the level of the ankle joint. As noted by Knupp and colleagues,[15] "the most important aspect of preoperative planning is assessment of the origin of the deformity." To identify the origin of the deformity, the surgeon must correctly locate the center or centers of rotation of angulation (CORA) and select the appropriate osteotomy for deformity correction.

A complete and thorough clinical and radiographic evaluation of the lower extremity from the hip through the foot is imperative for identifying all areas of rigid and reducible deformity. As part of the clinical evaluation, the deltoid and lateral ankle complexes should be stressed to determine the need for ligament release or reconstruction, and the Silfverskiöld test should be performed to determine

Table 1
Indications and contraindications

Indications	Contraindications
• Asymmetric ankle osteoarthritis with varus/valgus deformity and ≥50% preserved tibiotalar joint surface[25]	Absolute
	• End-stage ankle osteoarthritis with ≤50% preserved tibiotalar joint surface[15,25]
• Isolated osteochondral lesion of the medial/lateral tibiotalar joint[25]	• Unmanageable hindfoot instability[15,25]
• Physeal growth arrest[7,26]	• Acute/chronic infection[15,28]
• Tibial torsion[7,26]	• Severe vascular deficiency[15,25]
• Tibial fracture malunion[15]	• Severe neurologic deficiency[15,25]
• Realignment before total ankle arthroplasty[15,26]	• Neuropathic disorders[15,25]
• Tibiotalar arthrodesis malunion[7,15]	Relative
• Residual paralytic deformities[7,27]	• Patient noncompliance[25]
• Congenital talipes equinovarus sequelae[7,27]	• Patients >70 y of age[15,25]
• Rheumatoid ankle[27]	• Impaired bone quality of the distal tibia or talus[15,25]
• Hemophilic arthropathy[27]	• Tobacco use[15,25]
	• Insulin-dependent diabetes mellitus[15]
	• Chronic skin abnormalities or soft tissue defects

Data from Refs.[7,15,25–28]

the need for posterior muscle group lengthening.[7,26] Ankle and subtalar joint range of motion should also be evaluated for reducibility.[7,25] Given the normal 2:1 inversion-to-eversion ratio, the subtalar joint inherently accommodates correction with valgus-producing osteotomies.[26,29] Conversely, if the subtalar joint is rigid and cannot accommodate the correction, additional inframalleolar procedures may be required.

Bilateral, full-length, calibrated, weight-bearing radiographs should be obtained to evaluate potential limb length discrepancies and deformities of the hip, knee, femur, and foot.[4,15,26] Hindfoot alignment radiographs should also be performed to assess the tibial-calcaneal relationship and computed tomography scans should be performed to evaluate the extent of arthritic destruction.[4,15] A recently proposed algorithm by Knupp and colleagues[19] factors in key aspects of the clinical and radiographic examination to guide procedure selection (**Figs. 1** and **2**).

Identifying frontal plane deformity

The first step in deformity planning is to assess the proximal and distal joint orientation on an anterior-posterior radiograph of the lower leg. This assessment can be accomplished by drawing proximal and distal mid-diaphyseal lines and measuring the medial proximal tibial angle (MPTA) (normal = 87°, range = 85°–90°) and the lateral distal tibial angle (LDTA) (normal = 89°, range = 86°–92°) (**Fig. 3**).[30] If the mid-diaphyseal lines are collinear, no bony deformity exists within the tibia. If the mid-diaphyseal lines

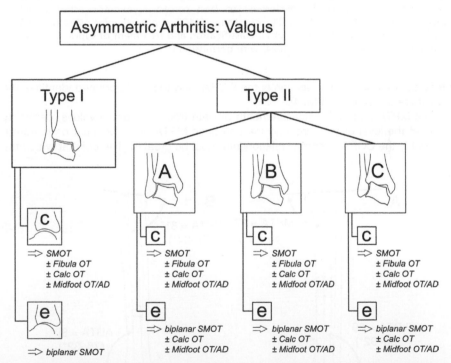

Fig. 1. Valgus asymmetric arthritis algorithm. This algorithm can be used to determine which procedures should be performed to best correct asymmetric arthritis with a valgus deformity. AD, arthrodesis; OT, osteotomy; SMOT, supramalleolar osteotomy. (*From* Knupp M, Stufkens SA, Bolliger L, et al. Classification and treatment of supramalleolar deformities. Foot Ankle Int 2011;32:1025; with permission.)

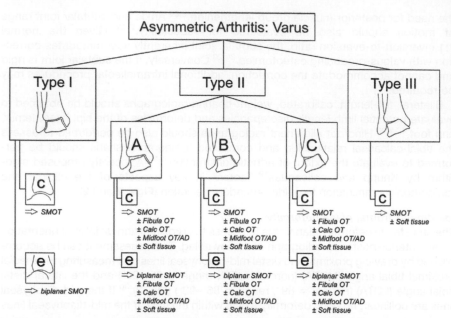

Fig. 2. Varus asymmetric arthritis algorithm. This algorithm can be used to determine which procedures should be performed to best correct asymmetric arthritis with a varus deformity. AD, arthrodesis; OT, osteotomy; SMOT, supramalleolar osteotomy. (*From* Knupp M, Stufkens SA, Bolliger L, et al. Classification and treatment of supramalleolar deformities. Foot Ankle Int 2011;32:1024; with permission.)

intersect, the point of intersection is the CORA, and the angle created identifies the magnitude of deformity (**Fig. 4**).

If the MPTA and LDTA measurements deviate from the normal values, deformity exists at the level of the joint, and the anatomic MPTA or LDTA must be restored. To identify the CORA, a normal relationship must be created. The point at which the

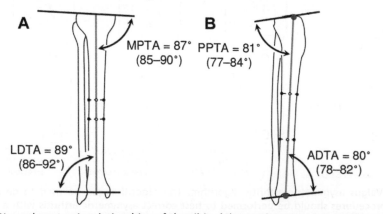

Fig. 3. Normal anatomic relationships of the tibia. (*A*) Anterior-posterior: MPTA and LDTA. (*B*) Lateral: PPTA and ADTA. (*Adapted from* Paley D. Principles of deformity correction. Berlin: Springer-Verlag; 2002. p. 9; with permission.)

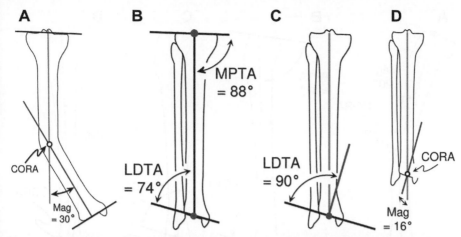

Fig. 4. Frontal plane deformity planning. (*A*) With normal proximal and distal joint relationships, mid-diaphyseal lines intersect identifying a CORA in the diaphysis with a magnitude of deformity of 30°. (*B*) With collinear mid-diaphyseal lines, a normal MPTA and an abnormal LDTA indicate a deformity at the distal joint line. The measured LDTA is less than the normal value indicating a valgus deformity. (*C*) A normal LDTA is drawn and (*D*) the point where it intersects the mechanical axis identifies a CORA with a magnitude of 16°. (*Adapted from* Paley D. Principles of deformity correction. Berlin: Springer-Verlag; 2002. p. 71, 76; with permission.)

normal angle intersects the mechanical axis represents the CORA. The angle defines the magnitude of the deformity (see **Fig. 4**). A varus deformity exists when the LDTA is greater than the normal range, and the reverse is true for a valgus deformity. Note that multiple deformities can exist within the tibia on the frontal plane. If an obvious deformity is present within the tibia and a CORA does not fall at the location of the deformity, a masked deformity exists and must be located.[30] In addition, multiple CORAs can be created and used to correct the deformity, as is often necessary in patients with rickets or Blount's disease.

Identifying sagittal plane deformity
When evaluating bony deformities in the sagittal plane, the mid-diaphyseal lines are drawn and the proximal and distal joint orientation is evaluated. The posterior proximal tibial angle (PPTA) (normal = 81°, range = 77°–84°) and the anterior distal tibial angle (ADTA) (normal = 80°, range 78°–82°) are measured (see **Fig. 3**).[30] If the mid-diaphyseal lines are collinear, no bony deformity exists within the tibia. If the mid-diaphyseal lines intersect, the point of intersection is the CORA, and the angle created identifies the magnitude of deformity (**Fig. 5**).

If the PPTA and ADTA measurements deviate from the normal values, deformity exists at the level of the joint, and the anatomic PPTA or ADTA must be restored. The CORA and the magnitude of the deformity are identified using the previously described methodology for frontal plane deformities (see **Fig. 5**). On the sagittal plane, the PPTA is drawn one-fifth of the way from anterior to posterior along the joint line, whereas the ADTA is drawn from the center of the ankle joint. A procurvatum deformity exists when the ADTA is greater than the normal range, and the reverse is true for a recurvatum deformity. As with frontal plane deformity planning, masked deformities must be identified.

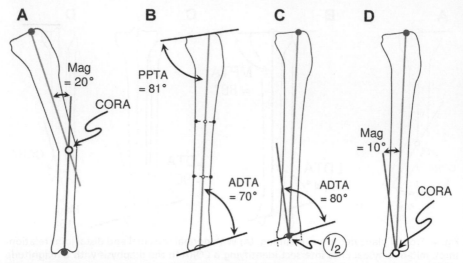

Fig. 5. Sagittal plane deformity planning. (*A*) With normal proximal and distal joint relationships, mid-diaphyseal lines intersect, identifying a CORA in the diaphysis with a magnitude of 20°. (*B*) Collinear mid-diaphyseal lines, a normal PPTA, and an abnormal ADTA indicate deformity at the distal joint line. The measured ADTA is less than the normal value indicating a recurvatum deformity. (*C*) A normal ADTA is drawn and (*D*) the point where it intersects the mechanical axis identifies a CORA with a magnitude of 10°. (*Adapted from* Paley D. Principles of deformity correction. Berlin: Springer-Verlag; 2002. p. 166; with permission.)

Osteotomy principles

Simply stated, an osteotomy performed at the location of CORA only requires angulation for reduction.[30] If the osteotomy is performed at a location other than the CORA, but the angulation correction axis (ACA) is located at the CORA, both angulation and translation are required for reduction.[30] The ACA is a point in space that represents the hinge around which the deformity is corrected. An osteotomy should not be created away from both CORA and ACA, because this will result in a secondary deformity and prohibit reduction.[30] When performing an osteotomy, if the ACA is located on the convex side of the bone, an opening wedge correction occurs. If the reverse is true, a closing wedge correction occurs (**Fig. 6**). In either scenario, the opposite cortex remains intact.[30] Osteotomies should always be made as close as possible to the level of the deformity to restore normal angles and realign the center of the ankle joint for proper biomechanical function.[28]

Performance of a fibular osteotomy

As a general rule, if identical deformities are located in the fibula and the tibia, an osteotomy should be performed at the same level in both bones.[30] Depending on the tibial deformity, one of the following osteotomy combinations should be selected:

1. Tibial and fibular opening wedge[30]
2. Tibial and fibular closing wedge[30]
3. Tibial opening wedge and fibular closing wedge[30]

When using a translation/angulation osteotomy, the fibula should be osteotomized slightly distal to the tibia. If there is no fibular deformity and the tibial deformity angulates the plafond toward the fibula, the fibula does not require an osteotomy, because it will not be affected during reduction.[30]

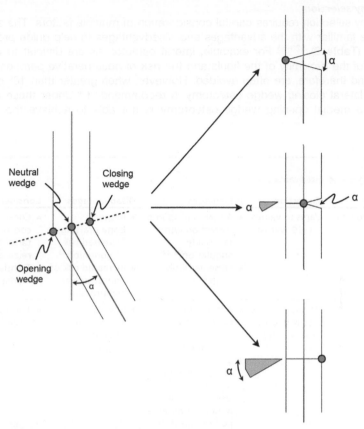

Fig. 6. Osteotomy selection. When the ACA is located on the convex side of the bone, an opening wedge correction occurs. When the ACA is located on the concave side, a closing wedge correction occurs. In addition, although rarely performed, a neutral wedge osteotomy can be created when the same degree of opening and closing would allow for deformity correction. The magnitude of correction is defined by α. (*Adapted from* Paley D. Principles of deformity correction. Berlin: Springer-Verlag; 2002. p. 102; with permission.)

Acute versus gradual correction

The decision to use acute versus gradual correction is based on a variety of factors, including, but not limited to, the location of deformity, bone quality, the degree of required correction, and the risk of neurovascular compromise. Acute correction with internal fixation is optimal in most cases and permits a one-stage procedure. Internal fixation is particularly useful when combined with an opening wedge osteotomy and insertion of bone graft. The fixation buttresses the graft into place while healing ensues.[7] Acute correction with external fixation can also be used to hold the correction static while bony healing takes place. Gradual correction is often performed with the use of a 6-axis external fixator. External fixation is particularly useful in complex deformities to protect vital neurovascular structures[7,18,30] and to perform simultaneous lengthening of the tibial segment.[7,31] It can also prove beneficial when there is a compromised soft tissue envelope,[31] when there is poor bone quality,[30] or when early weight-bearing is necessary.[31]

Osteotomy selection

Osteotomy selection requires careful consideration of multiple factors. The surgeon should be familiar with the advantages and disadvantages to help guide procedure selection (**Table 2**).[7,28–35] For example, lateral osteotomies are difficult to perform because of the proximity of the fibula and the risk of postoperative peroneal weakness,[27] and therefore, are often avoided. However, when greater than 10° of varus exists, a lateral closing wedge osteotomy is recommended.[4] Under these circumstances, a medial opening wedge osteotomy is not able to achieve the desired

Table 2
Advantages and disadvantages

Approach	Correction	Advantages	Disadvantages	Considerations
Medial opening wedge	Varus to valgus (<10° varus)	• Allows multiplane correction with saw blade angulation[29,32] • Preserves limb length[33,34]	• Requires bone grafting; increased risk of nonunion[33] • Increased risk of neurovascular compromise[33]	• Consider concomitant tarsal tunnel release[28,30] • Translation is medial[29]
Medial closing wedge	Valgus to varus (any degree deformity)	• Allows multiplane correction with saw blade angulation[29] • Decreased risk of neurovascular compromise[33] • Decreased risk of nonunion because no bone graft is used[35]	• Results in shortening of limb length[33]	• Translation is lateral[30]
Lateral closing wedge	Varus to valgus (>10° varus)	• Allows multiplane correction with saw blade angulation[29] • Decreased risk of nonunion because no bone graft is used[35]	—	• Translation is medial[30]
Focal dome	Valgus to varus OR varus to valgus	• Ideal for frontal/sagittal plane deformity with CORA at level of the ankle joint[29,31] or in the talus • Preserves limb length[7,28] • No thermal necrosis[28] • Minimal periosteal dissection[28] • Excellent bone to bone contact[28]	• Single-plane correction[29]	• Should be performed in metaphyseal bone[30]

Data from Refs.[7,28–35]

correction because the opening is restricted by the fibula.[4] Similarly, when correcting recurvatum/procurvatum deformities, posterior osteotomies are notoriously difficult to perform because of anatomic restrictions; therefore, anterior opening, anterior closing, and focal dome osteotomies are often selected. Recurvatum correction requires anterior translation, whereas procurvatum correction requires posterior translation. When feasible, all osteotomies should be made as distally as possible, preferably in the metaphysis to take advantage of metaphyseal healing properties while still allowing for adequate placement of internal fixation.[30] Note, deformity can exist in 2 planes and can be corrected by angulating the osteotomies cuts appropriately.

To optimize clinical results, concomitant procedures may be required.[19] For instance, when performing a varus or procurvatum correction that places tension along the neurovascular structures, a concomitant prophylactic tarsal tunnel release should be considered.[28,30] When presented with a limb length discrepancy and the operative limb is the shorter segment, closing wedge osteotomies should be avoided when possible to prevent additional shortening.[7,33,34]

Calculating the degree of deformity correction

During the stages of preoperative planning, it is imperative to calculate the extent of wedge resection or the quantity of bone graft needed to achieve the desired degree of correction. To calculate the desired degree of correction, a formerly established equation can be used.[25,34]

$$H = \tan \alpha_1 W$$

where H equals the height of the wedge to be resected or grafted, α_1 is the magnitude of deformity plus the degrees of overcorrection, and W equals the width of the tibia at the level of the osteotomy.[25,34] Using this equation results in a 1:1 ratio of degrees corrected to millimeters of wedge resection or grafting, up to 5 to 6 cm of correction.[34] Overcorrection between 2° and 5° is recommended.[9,11,36]

Preparation and Patient Positioning

Patient positioning must allow for sufficient exposure and access to the necessary anatomy and must avoid iatrogenic injury to the surrounding tendons and neurovascular structures. The specific position is dictated by the elected surgical approach (**Table 3**).

Surgical Approach

The surgical approach is selected based on the osteotomy necessary to correct the deformity and the need for fixation. It is important to evaluate the local soft tissue conditions and the presence of previous incisions or wounds. Maintaining an appropriate distance between areas of prior skin compromise will facilitate healing of surgical

Table 3 Patient positioning	
Surgical Approach	**Patient Positioning**
Anterior	Supine
Lateral	1. Lateral decubitus 2. Supine with sandbag under ipsilateral buttock
Medial	Supine with knee bent, sandbag under ipsilateral calf

incisions. General anesthesia is often used in conjunction with a regional anesthetic, but can be replaced with a solitary spinal anesthetic. The lower leg is exsanguinated with insufflation of a pneumatic tourniquet. Before incision, soft tissue and bony landmarks should be marked. Regardless of approach, care must be exercised during exposure of the tibia or fibula to avoid stripping of the periosteal layer, which could devascularize the osteotomy site.

Lateral approach
An 8- to 10-cm longitudinal incision is placed over the anterior margin of the distal fibula, which also provides access to the distal tibia. In some patients, an aberrant branch of the superficial peroneal nerve courses along the incision; therefore, caution should be used during dissection. Branches of the peroneal artery are normally encountered and should be cauterized as needed. Toward the distal aspect of the incision lies the anterior syndesmotic ligament, which can also be exposed, if necessary.

Medial approach
An 8- to 10-cm longitudinal incision is centered along the medial malleolus and carried proximally in line with the tibial crest. The saphenous nerve and vein are typically anterior to the incision, but branches may need to be addressed. A full-thickness flap is most reliable in avoiding injury to the anterior neurovascular structures. The sheath of the posterior tibial tendon is incised to allow posterior retraction of the tendon and visualization of the distal tibia.

Anterior approach
The incision is started over the ankle joint and extended proximally along the border of the anterior tibial crest. Traversing branches of the superficial peroneal nerve may be encountered along the distal portion of the incision. On exposure of the proximal extensor retinaculum, it is divided between the tibialis anterior and extensor hallucis longus tendons; exposure of the individual tendons should be avoided if at all possible. Deeper dissection is carried down between the tendons, with lateral retraction of the underlying neurovascular bundle. If surgical procedures within the ankle joint are anticipated, the overlying anterior capsule can be incised.

Surgical Procedure

Wedge osteotomy
Once adequate exposure of the tibia is achieved, soft tissue structures must be protected to avoid iatrogenic injury. Using fluoroscopy, a single K-wire is positioned parallel to the joint surface to act as a reference during correction. A series of K-wires can be placed based on preoperative planning for use as reference during the osteotomy. Before the osteotomy, care must be taken to ensure the proper placement of the wires and to avoid creating a secondary deformity. With use of a saw blade, the osteotomy is created using copious irrigation to avoid thermal injury to the bone. To avoid injury to the opposite cortex and soft tissue structures, the osteotomy can be completed with an osteotome. The far cortex should not be cut through the periosteal layer, but allowed to act as a hinge for the osteotomy to maintain stability. Preoperative and postoperative radiographs are shown in **Figs. 7** and **8**. With an opening wedge osteotomy, the material used for bone grafting is based on surgeon preference, patient characteristics, and the desired degree of correction.

Focal dome osteotomy
This osteotomy can performed open or percutaneously through a series of small stab incisions. For the open technique, once adequate exposure of the tibia is achieved, the

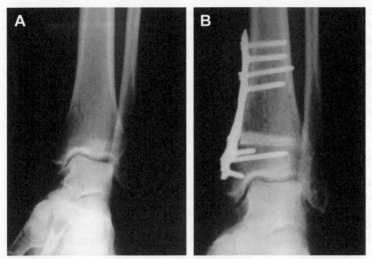

Fig. 7. Medial opening wedge tibial osteotomy. Patient presented with medial-based ankle pain. (*A*) There was radiographic evidence of varus angulation and medial joint space narrowing. (*B*) An opening wedge tibial osteotomy with placement of cortico-cancellous bulk wedge allograft was performed. Fixation was performed with locking medial tibial pilon plate.

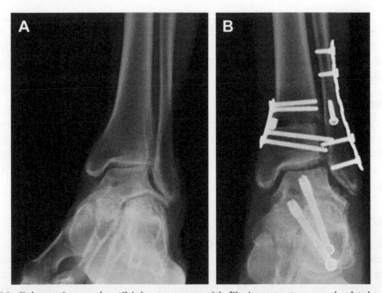

Fig. 8. Medial opening wedge tibial osteotomy with fibular osteotomy and subtalar fusion. Patient presented with pan-talar arthritis. (*A*) On weight-bearing radiographs, there was asymmetric joint space narrowing of the ankle. (*B*) An opening wedge tibial osteotomy with placement of medial-based opening wedge plate and cancellous chips with autograft was performed. A fibular osteotomy and subtalar fusion were also performed in the same setting to restore weight-bearing axis and to address posttraumatic arthritis.

neurovascular structures must be protected to avoid tensioning or tethering on the edges of the distal fragment. The cylindrical-shaped osteotomy can be created with several techniques. Most commonly, a single schanz pin is placed central and parallel to the joint in the frontal and sagittal planes to act as the point of rotation for the arched osteotomy. A focal dome osteotomy guide is placed over the pin, and a series of drill holes are created along the arc. Under fluoroscopic guidance, holes should be drilled from one cortex to the other. An osteotome or saw is used to connect the drill holes, completing the osteotomy. With the use of a saw blade, copious irrigation should be used to avoid thermal injury to the bone. The distal fragment is shifted to correct the deformity according to the preoperative plan. The schanz pin can be used to aid in positioning of the distal fragment before fixation.

Fibular osteotomy
Once adequate exposure of the fibula is achieved, soft tissue structures must be protected to avoid iatrogenic injury. Using fluoroscopy, the osteotomy is made in accordance with preoperative planning. As previously noted, when using a saw blade, copious irrigation can assist to avoid thermal injury to the bone.

Fixation of osteotomy
Fixation stability is vital to outcomes. Compared with standard plating techniques, locking plate technology provides a more rigid construct. However, locking plates do not make up for a lack of adherence to the general principles of osseous fixation. Compression through the osteotomy with a tensioning device can promote more reliable biological healing. When possible, interfragmentary fixation is recommended. Opening wedge osteotomies are generally not compressible, unless a corticocancellous bone graft is used.

Surgical Closure

After thorough irrigation of the incisions, layered closure is performed over a deep drain to avoid development of a hematoma. Primary closure of the tendon sheath or retinaculum will avoid instability of the tendons, but care must be taken to avoid overtightening.

Immediate Postoperative Care

A bulky Jones roll is incorporated into the surgical dressing to allow for compression. Provisional stability is achieved with a postoperative splint. Patients are strictly non-weight-bearing. If a deep drain is used, it is withdrawn within the first postoperative day. Sutures are removed between 2 and 3 weeks, based on the degree of soft tissue swelling.

REHABILITATION AND RECOVERY

Patients are non-weight-bearing immediately after surgery. Following their postoperative splint and dressing, a short leg non-weight-bearing cast is applied for 6 to 8 weeks until radiographic evidence of bony union is noted. Over the course of a month, patients are graduated to a progressive weight-bearing program within a walking boot. Once the cast is discontinued, a rehabilitation program is initiated, which includes range of motion, progressive strengthening, proprioception, and gait training. Functional improvement dictates transition back to full activity. Following surgery, full bony union is generally achieved within 3 to 6 months and complete functional recovery is often seen within 6 to 12 months.

CLINICAL RESULTS IN THE LITERATURE

In 1995, Takakura and colleagues[36] first introduced the low tibial osteotomy for the correction of asymmetric ankle joint arthritis. Most notably, the study found arthroscopic evidence of fibrocartilage formation, adding validity to their hypothesis that deformity correction and limb realignment shift the loading stress and slow the progression of ankle joint arthritis.[36] Since this preliminary investigation, several studies have provided clinical evidence demonstrating that the SMO consistently improves pain,[9–12,15,16,19,21–24] function,[9–12,14–24] and range of motion[9,11,13,15,22] with a low risk of complications (Table 4).[9–12,15–24,36–44]

Although the vast majority of evidence is limited to retrospective evaluation, prospective studies lend further validity to this technique. In 2008, Pagenstert and colleagues[22] conducted a prospective comparative evaluation and showed that, following realignment surgery, pain and function significantly improved with significant increases in sporting activity. However, the study also found an association between sporting activity and revision rate. Therefore, following realignment surgery, patients should be cautioned against frequent participation in high-impact sports that could increase

Table 4 Complications summary		
Complication	Count (%)	Range
Progression of OA requiring TAR	23 (3.0)	0–9
Progression of OA	9 (1.2)	0–4
Progression of OA requiring arthrodesis	9 (1.2)	0–3
Recurrent deformity/undercorrection/overcorrection	20 (2.6)	0–5
Nonunion	17 (2.2)	0–3
Persistent pain	17 (2.2)	0–7
Revision	14 (1.9)	0–7
Delayed union	9 (1.2)	0–4
Decreased range of motion	9 (1.2)	0–6
Removal of prominent implants	4 (0.5)	0–4
Pin site infection	31 (4.2)	0–3
Wound complication	19 (2.5)	0–6
Superficial infection	10 (1.3)	0–31
Deep/late infection	3 (0.4)	0–1
Tendon laceration requiring repair	4 (0.5)	0–3
Nerve damage	4 (0.5)	0–2
Scar complication	3 (0.4)	0–2
Fracture	3 (0.4)	0–3
Deep venous thrombosis	1 (0.1)	0–1
Compartment syndrome	1 (0.1)	0–1
Complex regional pain syndrome	1 (0.1)	0–1
Septic ankle arthritis	1 (0.1)	0–1
Sepsis	1 (0.1)	0–1

Based on the complications previously reported throughout the literature, a summary table was created. Articles written in any language other than English were excluded. A total of 23 studies and 758 ankles were included.
Abbreviation: OA, osteoarthritis.
Data from Refs.[9–12,15–24,36–44]

the risk of revision. In addition, in 2011, Knupp and colleagues[19] designed a prospective study that used an algorithm to determine which procedures should be performed concomitantly with the SMO. The study demonstrated significant improvements in pain and the American Orthopaedic Foot and Ankle Surgeon hindfoot scores, suggesting that additional procedures may be required to achieve a symmetrically loaded ankle joint.[19] Prospective and retrospective studies alike support the use of the SMO to achieve deformity correction with resultant reductions in pain and improved function.

Based on the information available, the risk of complications associated with the SMO is minimal (see **Table 4**).[9–12,15–24,36–44] Pin site infections are the most commonly reported, with one study reporting 27 of the 32 documented cases (84.4%),[18] followed by the progression of osteoarthritis requiring TAR, which affects approximately 3% of patients. Considering this finding, future studies should aim to identify risk factors that predispose patients to ankle joint deterioration, because this subset of patients may require an alternate surgical course. Recurrent deformity, undercorrection, and overcorrection are also frequently reported, further emphasizing the need for appropriate patient selection and thorough preoperative planning to achieve proper deformity correction.

In 2014, Colin and colleagues[5] conducted a retrospective comparison of talar positioning following SMO and TAR and found that anatomic hindfoot geometry is better restored following TAR. The authors credit the superior hindfoot geometry to the joint resurfacing and balancing procedures performed concomitantly with TAR.[5] With this information in mind, surgeons must carefully consider each patient. Some individuals, namely younger, more active patients, may be better suited for the joint-sparing SMO, which restores the mechanical axis of the tibia and permits conversion to a TAR later in life.

SUMMARY

The SMO should be considered a surgical treatment option for patients with beginning to midstage asymmetric ankle joint osteoarthritis and periarticular deformity. Studies have repetitively demonstrated that the SMO effectively achieves deformity correction, shifting the center of force and reducing peak pressures of the joint with resultant improvements in pain and functionality.[4–6,9–24] For optimal outcomes, however, surgeons must exercise appropriate patient selection, undergo meticulous preoperative planning, and execute the surgery with precision.

REFERENCES

1. Valderrabano V, Horisberger M, Russell I, et al. Etiology of ankle osteoarthritis. Clin Orthop Relat Res 2009;467:1800–6. Available at: http://www.ncbi.nlm.nih.gov/pmc/articles/PMC2690733/.
2. Saltzman CL, Salamon ML, Blanchard GM, et al. Epidemiology of ankle arthritis: report of a consecutive series of 639 patients from a tertiary orthopaedic center. Iowa Orthop J 2005;25:44–6. Available at: http://www.ncbi.nlm.nih.gov/pmc/articles/PMC1888779/.
3. Thomas RH, Daniels TR. Ankle arthritis. J Bone Joint Surg Am 2003;85-A:923–36. Available at: http://jbjs.org/content/85/5/923.long.
4. Barg A, Pagenstert GI, Horisberger M, et al. Supramalleolar osteotomies for degenerative joint disease of the ankle joint: indication, technique and results. Int Orthop 2013;37:1683–95. Available at: http://www.ncbi.nlm.nih.gov/pmc/articles/PMC3764298/.
5. Colin F, Bolliger L, Horn Lang T, et al. Effect of supramalleolar osteotomy and total ankle replacement on talar position in the varus osteoarthritic ankle: a

comparative study. Foot Ankle Int 2014;35:445–52. Available at: http://fai.sagepub.com/content/35/5/445.short.

6. Schmid T, Zurbriggen S, Zderic I, et al. Ankle joint pressure changes in a pes cavovarus model: supramalleolar valgus osteotomy versus lateralizing calcaneal osteotomy. Foot Ankle Int 2013;34:1190–7. Available at: http://fai.sagepub.com/content/34/9/1190.long.

7. Becker AS, Myerson MS. The indications and technique of supramalleolar osteotomy. Foot Ankle Clin 2009;14:549–61. Available at: http://www.sciencedirect.com/science/article/pii/S108375150900059X.

8. Giannini S, Buda R, Faldini C, et al. The treatment of severe posttraumatic arthritis of the ankle joint. J Bone Joint Surg Am 2007;89(Suppl 3):15–28. Available at: http://jbjs.org/content/89/suppl_3/15.

9. Pagenstert GI, Hintermann B, Barg A, et al. Realignment surgery as alternative treatment of varus and valgus ankle osteoarthritis. Clin Orthop Relat Res 2007; 462:156–68. Available at: http://journals.lww.com/corr/Abstract/2007/09000/Realignment_Surgery_as_Alternative_Treatment_of.25.aspx.

10. Tanaka Y, Takakura Y, Hayashi K, et al. Low tibial osteotomy for varus-type osteoarthritis of the ankle. J Bone Joint Surg Br 2006;88:909–13. Available at: http://www.bjj.boneandjoint.org.uk/content/88-B/7/909.full.

11. Cheng YM, Huang PJ, Hong SH, et al. Low tibial osteotomy for moderate ankle arthritis. Arch Orthop Trauma Surg 2001;121:355–8. Available at: http://link.springer.com/article/10.1007/s004020000243.

12. Colin F, Gaudot F, Odri G, et al. Supramalleolar osteotomy: techniques, indications and outcomes in a series of 83 cases. Orthop Traumatol Surg Res 2014; 100:413–8. Available at: http://www.sciencedirect.com/science/article/pii/S1877056814000784.

13. Kim YS, Park EH, Koh YG, et al. Supramalleolar osteotomy with bone marrow stimulation for varus ankle osteoarthritis: clinical results and second-look arthroscopic evaluation. Am J Sports Med 2014;42:1558–66. Available at: http://ajs.sagepub.com/content/early/2014/04/23/0363546514530669.abstract.

14. Ellington JK, Myerson MS. Surgical correction of the ball and socket ankle joint in the adult associated with a talonavicular tarsal coalition. Foot Ankle Int 2013;34: 1381–8. Available at: http://fai.sagepub.com/content/34/10/1381.

15. Knupp M, Barg A, Bolliger L, et al. Reconstructive surgery for overcorrected clubfoot in adults. J Bone Joint Surg Am 2012;94:e1101–7. Available at: http://jbjs.org/content/94/15/e110.

16. Mann HA, Filippi J, Myerson MS. Intra-articular opening medial tibial wedge osteotomy (plafond-plasty) for the treatment of intra-articular varus ankle arthritis and instability. Foot Ankle Int 2012;33:255–61. Available at: http://fai.sagepub.com/content/33/4/255.short.

17. Hintermann B, Barg A, Knupp M. Corrective supramalleolar osteotomy for malunited pronation-external rotation fractures of the ankle. J Bone Joint Surg Br 2011;93:1367–72. Available at: http://www.bjj.boneandjoint.org.uk/content/93-B/10/1367.abstract.

18. Horn DM, Fragomen AT, Rozbruch SR. Supramalleolar osteotomy using circular external fixation with six-axis deformity correction of the distal tibia. Foot Ankle Int 2011;32:986–93. Available at: http://fai.sagepub.com/content/32/10/986.short.

19. Knupp M, Stufkens SA, Bolliger L, et al. Classification and treatment of supramalleolar deformities. Foot Ankle Int 2011;32:1023–31. Available at: http://fai.sagepub.com/content/32/11/1023.short.

20. Lee WC, Moon JS, Lee K, et al. Indications for supramalleolar osteotomy in patients with ankle osteoarthritis and varus deformity. J Bone Joint Surg Am 2011; 93:1243–8. Available at: http://jbjs.org/content/93/13/1243.long.

21. Pagenstert G, Knupp M, Valderrabano V, et al. Realignment surgery for valgus ankle osteoarthritis. Oper Orthop Traumatol 2009;21:77–87. Available at: http://link.springer.com/article/10.1007%2Fs00064-009-1607-9.

22. Pagenstert G, Leumann A, Hintermann B, et al. Sports and recreation activity of varus and valgus ankle osteoarthritis before and after realignment surgery. Foot Ankle Int 2008;29:985–93. Available at: http://fai.sagepub.com/content/29/10/985.short.

23. Harstall R, Lehmann O, Krause F, et al. Supramalleolar lateral closing wedge osteotomy for the treatment of varus ankle arthrosis. Foot Ankle Int 2007;28:542–8. Available at: http://fai.sagepub.com/content/28/5/542.short.

24. Stamatis ED, Cooper PS, Myerson MS. Supramalleolar osteotomy for the treatment of distal tibial angular deformities and arthritis of the ankle joint. Foot Ankle Int 2003;24:754–64. Available at: http://fai.sagepub.com/content/24/10/754.short.

25. Barg A, Saltzman CL. Single-stage supramalleolar osteotomy for coronal plane deformity. Curr Rev Musculoskelet Med 2014;7:277–91. Available at: http://link.springer.com/article/10.1007%2Fs12178-014-9231-1.

26. Benthien RA, Myerson MS. Supramalleolar osteotomy for ankle deformity and arthritis. Foot Ankle Clin 2004;9:475–87 viii. Available at: http://www.sciencedirect.com/science/article/pii/S1083751504000518.

27. Tanaka Y. The concept of ankle joint preserving surgery: why does supramalleolar osteotomy work and how to decide when to do an osteotomy or joint replacement. Foot Ankle Clin 2012;17:545–53. Available at: http://www.sciencedirect.com/science/article/pii/S1083751512000563.

28. DiDomenico LA, Gatalyak N. End-stage ankle arthritis: arthrodiastasis, supramalleolar osteotomy, or arthrodesis? Clin Podiatr Med Surg 2012;29:391–412. Available at: http://www.sciencedirect.com/science/article/pii/S0891842212000523.

29. Rush SM. Supramalleolar osteotomy. Clin Podiatr Med Surg 2009;26:245–57. Available at: http://www.sciencedirect.com/science/article/pii/S0891842208001171.

30. Paley D. Principles of deformity correction. Berlin: Springer-Verlag; 2002.

31. Siddiqui NA, Herzenberg JE, Lamm BM. Supramalleolar osteotomy for realignment of the ankle joint. Clin Podiatr Med Surg 2012;29:465–82. Available at: http://www.sciencedirect.com/science/article/pii/S089184221200095X.

32. Mendicino RW, Catanzariti AR, Reeves CL. Percutaneous supramalleolar osteotomy for distal tibial (near articular) ankle deformities. J Am Podiatr Med Assoc 2005;95:72–84. Available at: http://www.japmaonline.org/doi/abs/10.7547/0950072.

33. Myerson MS, Zide JR. Management of varus ankle osteoarthritis with joint-preserving osteotomy. Foot Ankle Clin 2013;18:471–80. Available at: http://www.sciencedirect.com/science/article/pii/S1083751513000521.

34. Mangone PG. Distal tibial osteotomies for the treatment of foot and ankle disorders. Foot Ankle Clin 2001;6:583–97. Available at: http://www.sciencedirect.com/science/article/pii/S1083751503001153.

35. Stamatis ED, Myerson MS. Supramalleolar osteotomy: indications and technique. Foot Ankle Clin 2003;8:317–33. Available at: http://www.sciencedirect.com/science/article/pii/S1083751503000184.

36. Takakura Y, Tanaka Y, Kumai T, et al. Low tibial osteotomy for osteoarthritis of the ankle. Results of a new operation in 18 patients. J Bone Joint Surg Br 1995;77: 50–4. Available at: http://www.bjj.boneandjoint.org.uk/content/77-B/1/50.long.

37. de Roode CP, Hung M, Stevens PM. Supramalleolar osteotomy: a comparison of fixation methods. J Pediatr Orthop 2013;33:672–7. Available at: http://journals. lww.com/pedorthopaedics/Abstract/2013/09000/Supramalleolar_Osteotomy___A_ Comparison_of.16.aspx.

38. Eidelman M, Katzman A, Zaidman M, et al. Deformity correction using supramalleolar gigli saw osteotomy and Taylor spatial frame: how to perform this osteotomy safely? J Pediatr Orthop B 2011;20:318–22. Available at: http://journals.lww.com/ jpo-b/Abstract/2011/09000/Deformity_correction_using_supramalleolar_gigli.10. aspx.

39. Knupp M, Stufkens SA, Pagenstert GI, et al. Supramalleolar osteotomy for tibiotalar varus malalignment. Tech Foot Ankle Surg 2009;8:17–23. Available at: http:// journals.lww.com/techfootankle/Abstract/2009/03000/Supramalleolar_Osteotomy_ for_Tibiotalar_Varus.6.aspx.

40. Neumann HW, Lieske S, Schenk K. Supramalleolar, subtractive valgus osteotomy of the tibia in the management of ankle joint degeneration with varus deformity. Oper Orthop Traumatol 2007;19:511–26. Available at: http://europepmc.org/ abstract/med/18071935.

41. Best A, Daniels TR. Supramalleolar tibial osteotomy secured with the Puddu plate. Orthopedics 2006;29:537–40. Available at: http://www.healio.com/orthopedics/ journals/ortho/2006-6-29-6/%7Bfb353ed7-a0dc-4dbd-9705-99a79ed42289%7D/ supramalleolar-tibial-osteotomy-secured-with-the-puddu-plate.

42. Eidelman M, Bialik V, Katzman A. Correction of deformities in children using the Taylor spatial frame. J Pediatr Orthop B 2006;15:387–95. Available at: http:// journals.lww.com/jpo-b/Abstract/2006/11000/Correction_of_deformities_in_children_ using_the.1.aspx.

43. Takakura Y, Takaoka T, Tanaka Y, et al. Results of opening-wedge osteotomy for the treatment of a post-traumatic varus deformity of the ankle. J Bone Joint Surg Am 1998;80:213–8. Available at: http://jbjs.org/content/80/2/213.

44. Pearce MS, Smith MA, Savidge GF. Supramalleolar tibial osteotomy for haemophilic arthropathy of the ankle. J Bone Joint Surg Br 1994;76:947–50. Available at: http://www.bjj.boneandjoint.org.uk/content/76-B/6/947.short.

Index

Note: Page numbers of article titles are in **bold face** type.

Clin Podiatr Med Surg 32 (2015) 463–472
http://dx.doi.org/10.1016/S0891-8422(15)00038-5
0891-8422/15/$ – see front matter © 2015 Elsevier Inc. All rights reserved.

podiatric.theclinics.com